VEGAN NUTRITION

34 Experts Discuss

VLADIMIR KAY

Dedication

To all the vegans who might have missed
some key nutritional advice that is needed
in order to make their lives healthy and happy.

Acknowledgements

Thank you to all the people who
generously agreed to contribute to this book.

Table of Contents

Introduction

When I was growing up and during my college years and early working life, I ate what is referred to as the standard American diet—excessive amounts of protein, processed grains, and carbohydrates with added sugars. Then for four years, while traveling almost constantly for a management consulting firm, I usually ate in three different restaurants every day in addition to eating again late at night after work. It was a highly stressful period in my life. I didn't eat junk food and I never ate French fries, or white bread, or greasy hamburgers. I ate expensive steaks, sushi, and many kinds of fine cheese. I thought that what I ate was healthy but I was eating a lot of food and, in hindsight, a lot of what I ate was protein.

One day, I began to question my lifestyle and the huge amount of food I was eating. I thought that all of that food couldn't be healthy, so, I started doing some research. I looked at some documentaries about food and read some books about food. I began to think that there must be a connection between the diet one eats and the health of the world ecosystem. I started experimenting with different diets and I learned how the food we eat affects our bodies. Eventually, I came to the decision that a vegan diet would be a healthy choice for me, and I liked the fact that I would not be eating animals that came from confined and unhealthy feeding operations.

When I started my vegan lifestyle, I thought I had a good understanding of it. I ate a lot of vegetables and salads and I was careful in following the diet. I thought that being vegan would be an excellent life choice. For nutritional reasons, I thought that going either completely plant based or very close to it would be healthy. The health-promoting properties of the nutrients in plants have long been known, and these properties have been documented in the scientific and medical communities.

Unfortunately, however, I did not understand a few key vegan concepts and that resulted in a number of nutritional and psychological imbalances. After eight months of following a strict vegan diet, I suffered some very uncomfortable consequences including a severe vitamin deficiency and an uncharacteristic fatigue and moodiness.

Something wasn't right, but I couldn't find the answers anywhere for how I felt. I didn't want to rely on information I could find on the internet and I didn't want to rely on just a few people I could talk with. Most people have a slightly unique interpretation of facts and they also have personal biases, so, it's not prudent to rely on just one or even just a few expert opinions. I decided I would try to talk with as many nutritionists in the country that I could find. I thought that would be the only way I could understand how I was feeling.

Over time, I personally interviewed more than fifty experts in nutrition. Some of these experts are famous in the field of nutrition, such as Dr. Marion Nestle and Dr. Colin Campbell. Some are professors in elite institutions and others are nutritionists with decades of hands-on experience treating patients. All of them have something interesting and counterintuitive to say. All are experts on nutrition first, and vegan nutrition second. General nutrition experts were prioritized over die-hard vegan nutritionists in an effort to avoid the tendency to interpret new evidence as confirmation of one's existing beliefs or theories.

Not surprisingly, there are a few things that these experts disagree with, but there is an overwhelming majority of things that all of them do agree with. This book is a collection of my interviews and I found answers to how I was feeling after a strict vegan diet. One of the things I learned is that any extreme diet poses risks, and that includes veganism, although a diet totally of plants seems safer than some other extreme diets such as the grapefruit diet. I encourage you, the reader, to find food patterns for yourself, and to think carefully about them.

My hope is that this book will give you some ideas to experiment with and that you might refine your diet and lifestyle until you are living the healthiest and happiest life possible.

Marion Nestle

Dr. Nestle is the Paulette Goddard Professor of Nutrition, Food Studies, and Public Health Emerita at New York University, which she chaired from 1988 to 2003 and from which she officially retired in September 2017. She is also a Visiting Professor of Nutritional Sciences at Cornell. She earned a Ph.D. in molecular biology and an MPH in public health nutrition from the University of California, Berkeley, and has been awarded honorary degrees from Transylvania University in Kentucky (2012) and from the City University of New York's Macaulay Honors College (2016).

Top quote

Nutrition advice is so simple that Michael Pollan does it in seven words: "Eat food. Not too much. Mostly plants."

What book about nutrition do you frequently recommend to friends?

My own, of course! *Food Politics,* for those interested. *What to Eat,* for basic issues about nutrition. *Eat, Drink, Vote* (a cartoon book), for food politics "lite." *Why Calories Count,* for information about calories and energy balance. *Soda Politics,* for people interested in advocating for less sugar in beverages. *Unsavory Truth,* for explanations of how food companies influence science.

What are the top risks of a vegan diet that you've seen, and how would you recommend avoiding those risks?

Not eating a variety, not eating enough calories, eating too many calories, not getting vitamin B12.

Three big meals or seven small meals?
I don't think it matters. It's the overall calories that matter.

What purchase of fifty dollars or less has improved your ability to follow a healthy diet the most?
A bathroom scale.

What are the two foods you'd recommend to stop eating or drastically cut out?
I think it's possible and desirable to eat foods you like, whatever they are, in reasonable amounts.

What is the worst advice you hear people give routinely in the nutrition community?
Sometimes I hear that nutrition is so confusing that you don't have to pay attention to it. Actually, nutrition advice is so simple that Michael Pollan does it in seven words: "Eat food. Not too much. Mostly plants."

Low-fat vs. low-carb diet for weight loss?
I don't think it matters. The overall calories matter the most for weight.

Is there a superfood that you recommend?
I don't believe there is such a thing as a superfood.

Breakfast or no breakfast?
Whichever you prefer.

What is detoxification, including intermittent fasting, and how do you feel about the need for it?
The body detoxifies itself. Nothing else is needed.

In the past few years, what attitude or belief has shaped your understanding of healthy nutrition and lifestyle the most?
My views have been consistent since the mid-1970s when I first studied nutrition.

What do you do when you're craving junk food?
Eat it. Just not too much.

Dayong Wu

Dr. Dayong Wu is a scientist and an Associate Director at the Nutritional Immunology Laboratory at the Human Nutrition Research Center on Aging. His research interests include age-related changes in immune cells; the effects of nutrients, dietary components, and functional food on immune and inflammatory responses; and autoimmune disorders. Dr. Wu is an Associate Professor of Nutrition at the Friedman School of Nutrition Science and Policy at Tufts University. He is a member of the American Society for Nutritional Sciences as well as the American Aging Association.

Top quote

"Limiting cholesterol no longer makes sense and saturated fats are at least neutral, not harmful."

What book about nutrition do you frequently recommend to friends and clients?

I personally like *Eat, Drink, and be Healthy: the Harvard Medical School Guide to Healthy Eating* by Walter Willet, and *What to Eat* by Marion Nestle. What they talked about is based on science, not anecdote, and they have broad knowledge in both nutrition and public health as well as public policy.

How much does diet really affect mood and psychological well-being?

Theoretically, many nutrients and food components can provide substance for synthesizing molecules (like serotonin and its precursor tryptophan) that are known to favorably affect mood.

However, interventional studies have generated inconsistent results, for the large part. Although psychological well-being is quite subjective for assessment, psychological factors cannot be ruled out when an individual believes what he or she eats is supposed to be good or not.

What kind of diet or lifestyle is the most effective at preventing aging?

It definitely involves a multifactorial approach. An appropriate total energy intake and a balanced diet pattern are key factors. Having a total calorie intake to maintain a body weight within a normal range is important. Macronutrients should include protein, fat, and carbohydrates instead of pushing to the extreme in favor of one like the current trends for protein or fat.

Of course, carbs should come from complex forms like whole grains and fruits, instead of simple forms like sugary drinks and refined flour which basically are empty calories. Increased intake of fruits and vegetables is important in preventing many age-related chronic diseases; in particular, the metabolic diseases such as cardiovascular disease, Type 2 diabetes, and maybe neurodegenerative disease as well. For life style, there is nothing new. One should avoid smoking and practice moderate drinking, regular exercise, and active social communication in addition to maintaining interests in many things such as nature, social events, hobbies, etc.).

What are the two foods you'd recommend stopping eating or drastically cut out?

I don't think there is any food to be strictly forbidden, but we should cut down on sweets and keep fried food to a minimum. Fried food contains lots of calories, less nutrients because they are destroyed by high temperatures, and oils that are often repeatedly used and can accumulate to make unhealthy products which is otherwise low or non-existent in fresh oil.

What is the worst advice you hear people routinely give in the nutrition community?

"Don't eat meat," and "Don't drink milk," because they might increase your risk of developing cancers.

Low-fat vs. low-carb diet for weight loss?

Calorie is calorie, no matter where it is from. The low-fat strategy in the past decades has failed to reduce weight in the population and that is mainly due to the calorie income being shifted to carb. However, fats in food usually more efficiently increase satiety than carb-heavy food. In contrast, after consuming simple carb (high glycemic carb), one can more quickly feel hungry and, more importantly, it induces rapid insulin secretion, which is believed to be a risk factor for glucose intolerance and insulin resistance.

What is detoxification and how do you feel about the need for it?

Caloric restriction has been proposed to have a variety of health benefits. I have no knowledge about the comparison between general calorie restriction and intermittent fasting. I don't believe in the detoxification practice. Maybe it is just a matter of difference in what is meant by the concept, or different definitions, of "detoxification." So, if the "detoxification" suggests an increase in the consumption of fruits and vegetables, I would agree. But the health benefit is mainly from the fact that fruits and vegetables contain low calories, high fiber, high nutrients (vitamins, minerals), and high antioxidant phytochemicals. Fruits and vegetables can also increase the variety of gut microbiota and favorably modulate the composition of microbiota.

Breakfast or no breakfast?

We should have regular breakfast. A recent study showed that skipping breakfast did not help reduce weight but, rather, it did the opposite.

In the past few years, what new attitude or belief has most shaped your understanding of healthy nutrition and a healthy lifestyle?

The most dramatic change in our understanding of healthy is perhaps in fat. Specifically, limiting cholesterol no longer makes sense, and saturated fats are at least neutral, not harmful. Some studies have shown that whole milk is even better than low-fat milk in terms of metabolic health and weight control

Vladimir Kirichenko

William Masters

Dr. Masters is an economist in the Nutrition Department of Tufts University. He uses nutrition science to create an understanding of individual behavior and societal outcomes. He did his undergraduate studies at Yale University, and received a Ph.D. at the Food Research Institute At Stanford.

Top quote

"There is abundant evidence that mental state and physical energy are closely related but many other factors also contribute to mental health. In my limited experience, poor diet has not been the original cause of disorders. The original cause is something else."

What book about nutrition do you frequently recommend to friends?

My Year of Meats, by Ruth Ozeki. It's fun and insightful, unlike so much that's written about food. If people really want to learn about nutrition science, the profession's standard entry-level textbook, Wardlaw's *Contemporary Nutrition*, is actually quite readable.

How much does diet really affect mood and psychological well-being?

A lot. There is abundant evidence that mental state and physical energy are closely related. But many other factors also contribute to mental health - and in my limited experience, poor diet was not the original cause of disorders. The original cause was something else. Changes in appetite are important symptoms of many problems and, once diet quality worsens, it may be hard to recover.

Is the vegan diet equally good for everyone? Why or why not?

No, I see no reason why everyone "should" be vegan, but many people now eat too much red and processed meat relative to a healthy diet. The most recent instance of this argument is the EAT-Lancet report led by Walter Willett who is the world champion of this view. Another reason to limit animal foods is that livestock are often treated in terrible ways that are unacceptable to many people, including me. There is also evidence that many animal production systems cause environmental harm, e.g., methane burps of cows and other ruminants, and the land used to grow feed which would otherwise be used in other ways, as well as antibiotic resistance in settings where antibiotics for livestock are overused.

Nevertheless, none of those harms provide a persuasive call for zero anything. Ultimately, it's pretty clear that the evidence favors a flexitarian approach, in which choices depend on local circumstances at each place and time.

In my view, the only explanation or justification for zero is that some people prefer absolute rules, and a few people's absolute rules help nudge others to improve towards a balanced approach. A reducetarian, or flexitarian approach, with some red meat, poultry or pork, and milk and eggs can easily be helpful. These food groups are needed for human health especially in utero and infancy for maternal and child health, and they are useful in agriculture for crop-livestock interactions. Even animal welfare does not call for zero farmed animals, since that argument would rely on an ethical argument that places any suffering above the value of coming to life in the first place. Also, a big challenge ahead is how to limit harmful aspects of animal agriculture and other parts of the food system, while still helping poorer people get more of what they want and need. It's not helpful to focus entirely on only the diets of rich people, without focusing on what we can do to bring better diets into the reach of poorer people.

What are the top dangers of veganism, and how would you recommend avoiding them? More generally, what are the things that keep people from having a healthy, balanced, and sustainable diet?

As far as I can tell, the main danger associated with veganism is sanctimony, real or perceived. Whenever one group casts itself as enlightened, others will push back, and proponents will get stuck in an echo chamber. Some people are very skilled at pursuing their own ideals without losing contact with others. A great example of this for veganism is Ezra Klein, for instance, like in his memorable interview with Melanie Joy.

Three big meals or seven small meals? A lot of people are confused about snacking.

I don't know about meal size, as such, but intermittent fasting seems like one of the most exciting new frontiers in nutrition. Allowing for more complete digestion of everything one has eaten, especially overnight, could be a good idea for many reasons. I'm not sure the term "fasting" is the right word, however. I'd rather just call it concentrated mealtimes, choosing times when one can plan ahead for mindful eating.

What purchase of fifty dollars or less has improved your ability the most to have a healthy diet?

A bathroom scale. I step on it most days at about the same time and ignore small fluctuations, but I try to respond quickly to changes of more than a few pounds.

What are the two foods you'd recommend to stop eating or drastically cut out?

I wouldn't ban any one food, let alone two. Ingredients are another matter. One priority for global health is to spread the ban on trans fats to developing countries like India.

What is worst advice you hear people give routinely in the nutrition community?

There's too much noise, and no need to single out anything in particular.

What's the top "superfood" or supplement you recommend that everyone should incorporate into their diet?

There's nothing I would recommend to everyone. I happen to love peanut butter, but maybe that's because it was a favorite after-school snack when I was little. It was also handmade by villagers in rural Zimbabwe where I lived after college.

What is detoxification and how do you feel about the need for it or intermittent fasting?

I'm no expert on anything biochemical but I have seen some evidence suggesting that autophagy, triggered by periods of not eating, can be helpful. What I don't understand is why that is called detoxification. Why not just call it healthy metabolism?

Breakfast or no breakfast?

Presumably, that depends on the rest of one's daily schedule and family circumstances. I'm lucky and can choose my mealtimes, but many people don't have that luxury.

In the past few years, what new attitude or belief has most shaped your understanding of healthy nutrition and a healthy lifestyle?

There have been so many changes. New evidence has changed my understanding about a lot of things: lower carbs and more whole grains, healthier fats, concentrated meal times, exercise to avoid back pain, etc., but maybe those changes just trace my own aging.

What do you do when you're craving junk food?

I eat some and then stop. I'm an economist and one of our most important recurring themes is diminishing returns. The first few mouthfuls are the best tasting, and eventually one reaches the point where the harms outweigh the benefits. Economics is all about such U-shaped functions. That helps us learn when to stop, and being an economist might also have helped me to resist food marketing. A lot of what we find delicious is the power of suggestion.

Stan Kubow

Dr. Kubow obtained his Ph.D. in 1984 from the University of Guelph after obtaining undergraduate and graduate degrees at McGill University and the University of Toronto. He carried out postdoctoral studies at the University of Guelph and the University of Toronto from 1984 to 1987 prior to joining the School of Dietetics and Human Nutrition at McGill University as an Assistant Professor in 1987. He has been an Associate Professor since 1993 and he also served as Acting Director from 1993 to 1994. He serves on the editorial boards of Journal of Lipids, Nutrition and Medicine, and Journal of Nutrition and Metabolism. His daughter is vegan.

Top Quote

"One missing element in many discussions is what is optimal functionality?"

What book about nutrition do you frequently recommend to friends?

I never recommend a book because it's very hard to get a book that will cover everything. Also, often you have books with a single point of view that's highly biased and can confuse readers because it doesn't present the big picture. I actually don't use textbooks in my own course, because I try to cover the latest information. The field is evolving, so, usually when I teach I cover the nuances so that the latest research is covered.

Is the vegan diet equally good for everyone?
That is an interesting question. There isn't such thing as a vegan diet because it's not one diet. Based on the research and surveys, there's quite a cross section of vegan diets that are out there, from vegan diets that are focused on more processed foods, which are likely to have nutritional deficiencies, to those that have whole foods with lots of considerations.

As for whether some form of a vegan diet can be equally good for everyone, it depends on how much time you have to spend on considering and planning your diet. If it's a low-income family with children, and they have to feed them in a cost-effective and practical way, without expensive supplements and spending lots of time optimizing the various foods, then it's probably not a good idea.

If someone has lots of time and can consider all the parameters, and take tests to guard against deficiencies, it could be done.

Another key point is that there must be nutrition knowledge in order to follow a vegan diet correctly. There must be a thorough understanding of human nutritional needs and the various qualities of foods.

Considering all of this, I would say that it's not equally good for everyone.

What are the top risks of a vegan diet that you've seen, and how would you recommend avoiding those risks?
This question requires a thorough response. I will break it down into broader categories.

1. Overall
There are some misconceptions that the vegan diet leads to a healthy diet. You can have a healthy plant-based diet, but it doesn't necessarily mean that it's inherently healthier even if it's optimized. And actually, there are plenty of challenges associated with the vegan diet and key life phases, which we'll get into.

There are inherent benefits to having plant-based foods. The data is strong that consuming plant-based foods lowers the risk of non-communicable disease (metabolic disorders, chronic diseases, diabetes, etc.) There are a lot of health benefits associated with components in plant foods (carotenoids, polyphenols, etc.) All of these are plant-based food components that clearly have some protective effects against those diseases. The data is pretty persuasive that being vegan would give you the higher benefits associated with those foods versus a diet that is omnivore-centered and does not contain much plant-based food.

However, an omnivore diet that has lots of plant foods can have potentially the same benefits that are attributed to the plant-based components.

There's nothing in my mind that is magical about the vegan diet apart from the fact that you'll have more plant-based nutrients (also called phytochemicals). Typically, world-wide vegetable consumption is subpar. Depending on the study, with anywhere from six to twelve servings of vegetables a day, you start to get the benefits of these phytochemicals.

If you're vegan, you're not going to be consuming two of the big risks for the omnivore diet. First, you're avoiding processed meats. Processed meats contain nitrates, too much sodium, are cooked at a high temperature, etc., resulting in a variety of risks being associated with them. Second, you're not being exposed to some of the risk of red meat.

On the other hand, a vegan won't be exposed to some of the benefits of the omnivore diet, so, it's not a one-way flow of benefits.

For example, it was recently made clear that there are actually benefits to dairy fat that are protective against diabetes and obesity. The mechanisms still aren't clear, but there are clearly some compounds to dairy that have these protective benefits. Also, there are probiotics in dairy, which is another benefit.

Another example is that there are elements in fish that are clearly associated with benefits. Omega-3s in fish are associated with strong protective elements in an optimal diet. This is another thing that vegans won't benefit from.

These are just a few examples. There are others.

2. Risks by life phases

It's worth discussing some nutritional risks that are shared by vegans and the rest of the population. I teach nutrition through phases of life and looking at risks for each phase is a helpful way to look at a diet's ability to meet fundamental human needs. I look at the phases of pre-conception and pregnancy, lactation, early infancy, childhood, adulthood, and the elderly. In each of these phases, risks that are inherent to the general population are also applicable to the vegan population. The vegan diet is no protector against the major risks for all of these populations, and actually some of these major nutritional risks are enhanced in the vegan lifestyle.

3. Pregnancy

During pregnancy, iron deficiency is a prevalent condition. There are additional risks in the pregnancy phase, vegan or not.

Vitamin B12 is a big risk. Right now, abundant sources of folic acid are considered one of the major pros of the vegan diet. However, what is emerging is that too much folic acid with not enough B12 can affect which genes are being modified and expressed (turned on and off). Consequentially, what happens in pregnancy can have a bearing on future disease risk with multigenerational effects (particular expressions of genes can be turned on and continued on for future generations.) Because vegans are more at risk for B12 deficiency, this is an area of concern.

There are also some suggestions that the plant-based ALA Omega-3s aren't optimal for humans, either. It's generally accepted that most of the health attributes from Omega-3s come from the long-chain fatty acids (DHA). On the other hand, it's still unclear whether there have been negative health consequences associated with not enough DHA. In a related example, for children in an enriched environment, (an environment with lots of mental stimulation and the opposite to a lower income, inner-city type of environment), these effects can be mitigated. If the children are in a non-enriched environment, there could be negative effects associated with DHA shortages. So, the effects in pregnancy are still not clear.

Another key risk during pregnancy is lack of iodine. Vegans tend to eat natural salts that aren't iodized, and they tend to be iodine deficient. If people eat kelp supplements, that can also be dangerous because sometimes they can have too little or too much iodine, as there's a high degree of variation. One of the leading causes of cognitive dysfunctions in newborn children is iodine deficiency and this certainly affects brain function in adulthood as well. So, there's that risk factor for vegans, as well, and again, vegans are a high-risk group for iodine deficiency.

This last risk raises an important point. Things can be very nuanced if you're a vegan individual. If you're a salt-sensitive individual, you can't eat a lot of salt. Then you're at risk for iodine deficiency. At that point, you almost need a nutritionist. Things can become problematic. I don't think that the general population realizes that the avoidance of animal-based protein is not a sufficient heuristic and that, for most individuals, careful planning cannot be avoided.

4. Lactation

I'll keep it short here. A vegan Omega-6-rich diet tends to produce the fatty acids that are most associated with the Omega-3s. There's no persuasive data that this has major functional differences, but it's a compositional difference and more research is needed.

In the typical vegan diet, there's just not enough Omega-3s in general. The other key point is, again, lack of vitamin B12. We'll talk about this more below, but the important thing is that a typical B12 supplement may not be enough for everyone given absorption differences.

5. Infancy and childhood

The data does suggest that there's no major impact from a vegan lifestyle except slightly smaller stature. That may be due to elements such as zinc. Boys tend to be more at risk for zinc deficiency than girls. A study showed that boys who had biomarkers of zinc deficiency had slightly stunted growth. It's also important to differentiate not just the amount of zinc consumed, but how much of it is absorbed.

Zinc deficiency and Vitamin D deficiency can result in rickets. When you eliminate milk as a source of Vitamin D, which is fortified, you have to replace it somehow. Interestingly, even in southern latitudes, you have a prevalence of Vitamin D deficiency, and that's just in the general population. Vegans will be even more at risk. When you talk about other minerals and elements, there are potentially more risks.

The same thing holds for calcium. The great majority of the population isn't getting enough calcium. In fact, because the idea that lowering fat is good was taken in by general public health programs, there was a gradual elimination of milk and actually that affected bone mineral density. These changes in milk consumption have been associated with mineral bone density. Girls are at even greater risk, and that's a concern, because a large portion of bone mass is acquired at adolescence, which can put you at risk for osteoporosis. In fact, osteoporosis is considered a pediatric disease because of this.

There have been studies that show that dairy consumed in adolescence is associated with higher bone density. Bone health is one of the key issues in the pediatric population. Obviously, this is especially a concern for vegans.

Iron is an important issue, as well. It's important in infancy, in particular, because iron is related to brain growth. The data is pretty compelling that, if there's insufficient iron intake, there can be irreparable damage because the brain grows so quickly during infancy. In the vegan construct, the bioavailability of iron is low in general, so there's more risk.

The bioavailability of iron isn't great in supplements, so, the public recommendations have changed to actually move away from iron supplements and move towards natural sources, meat in particular.

It's kind of an interesting picture with vegans because, again, there are wonderful benefits of phytonutrients but you have to be really careful in balancing against the deficiencies. And, once more, the bioavailability of many of these nutrients, such as iron, is much lower in a vegan diet.

One last point about adolescence. With any kind of health obsession, it can make the caregivers obsessed and they lose clarity and objectivity. A common cause for the inadequate development of children is when their parents try to put them on any strict diet, which can have permanent negative effects (not just veganism, but any strict diet in general). This is an important risk for all caregivers to be aware of, and they should opt for more diversity in the diet, and rely on the body to get what it needs.

6. Adulthood

It's a very interesting scenario because there are health benefits and health risks. What's happening is the realization that vitamin B12 has some quite important benefits for health, particularly in the context of higher folic acid intake.

Of course, plant-food based diets generally have consistent protective elements against metabolic diseases. One has to look at the diet as a whole. If it's, for instance, containing more white rice or other refined grains, it may not have enough protective benefits and it might be more deleterious. Basically, if there's an abundance of processed and refined foods, they will not have the protective phytonutrients.

The other question is that a lot of the research studies mortality. Another question is what is "optimal for health" (mental health, physical health, etc.)? And this is still a big question.

Generally, people aren't aware that sub-clinical or mild nutritional deficiencies can impact cognitive health and physical health. If you're having a vegan diet, you could be mildly deficient in B12 or iron, and that would certainly be sub-optimal.

Regarding supplements, essentially, it's thought that if you're eating a plant food diet, the availability of key micro nutrients is lower. Some of these components may not be released or be available in plant-foods, so they won't be broken down. (Usually, in animal foods, the bioavailability improves.) B12 is an exception. People over the age of sixty, in general, should have a supplement source of B12 because after that age, even B12 from animal protein isn't well absorbed because gastric acid production decreases.

To be clear, with careful supplementation, vegan diets can avoid any micro-nutrient associated risk. However, it's important to take tests to make sure that you're meeting the right daily requirements.

Vitamin B12, in particular, often won't show any signs and symptoms, which will cause irreversible nerve damage.

You asked specifically about white rice and soy.

Regarding white rice, there has been consistency with population studies that white rice is a high glycemic food. The risks associated with white rice are consistent. Brown rice is definitely healthier. Some of the "negative" things associated with brown rice phytates are actually beneficial to gut health, so, it's hands down the healthier choice.

Regarding soy, the Isoflavones are an overly hyped negative aspect of soy. The estrogen-like quality of Isoflavones may be a factor if you're consuming very heavy amounts of soy. As always with nutrition, variety is key. You have benefits of a synergy of all the components that you consume, without any drawbacks. I generally have not seen good evidence for the risk for soy, particularly if you have a fortified source, for vegans.

In the past few years, what attitude or belief has most shaped your understanding of healthy nutrition and a healthy lifestyle?

One missing element in many discussions is, "What is optimal functionality?" Part of that is because there's a lack of tools to measure it in terms of physical performance, mental performance, mood, etc.

This is something that needs more attention in optimal health. Sure, it's important to assess risks and benefits of long-term lifespan and disease states, but a more granular investigation is needed to investigate the concept of optimal health.

There are many components here that can be optimized in any diet, be it vegan, omnivore, etc. The focus on diet alone doesn't lead to a clear picture. It's a triumvirate of diet, physical activity, and social health.

Social health is really underestimated. We are all social beings, and that's part of the reason why many people choose a particular diet, to be part of "a group." A social construct is emerging when you look at centenarians and healthy people.

It is generally very important for overall health for people to be part of a social construct. There is something then that happens to the brain. Anything to mitigate the effects of stress can really play an important role in overall health, and a healthy social life is certainly part of that.

Another example is that people who engage in group physical activities tend to engender better health outcomes than people who work out on their own.

Another aspect is an array of mental activities, such as mindfulness, prayer, etc., which work on the brain and contribute to health as well.

There's a very interesting connection, which is how all of these areas interact on gut health and on the microbiome. There's a strong interplay on the gut microbiome with all of these activities. There's crosstalk between factors that are released in your gut that affect your body, and things that your body does that affect the microbiome. This crosstalk, in particular, is an area of research that I'm focusing on. So, the microbes are significantly affected by what happens in your life. A hypothesis that I have is that mindfulness affects your microbiome.

There also may be sex differences underlying everything, which are under-researched. This is actually potentially a big modifier in terms of optimal health. This could be because women need higher amounts of iron than males due to blood loss, and it's harder to meet that on a vegan diet. There could be other reasons.

The key realization is that a holistic perspective is needed. It's an interplay of many factors: the microbiome, the social life, the diet, the exercise, etc. Overall health is almost like a footstool. You can't ignore any of the elements, and I would encourage people to examine where it is they can see the most improvement and then focus on that. The problem is that a lot of these effects can be subtle. You can ignore them, but subtle effects can have long-term consequences. Studies show that even a mild vitamin C deficiency can affect your reflexes and response times. Or you can have a great diet but, if you don't exercise enough, your organs will deteriorate because, if you don't use it, you lose it. Most of these factors are subtle and people aren't clearly motivated to act on any one of these things.

Deirdre Kay Tobias

Dr. Deirdre Tobias is an associate epidemiologist in the Brigham and Women's Hospital Department of Medicine's Division of Preventive Medicine and an Instructor at Harvard Medical School. Dr. Tobias received her doctorate in nutrition and epidemiology from the Harvard TH Chan School of Public Health. Her primary research interests include identifying lifestyle risk factors for prevention of obesity-related chronic diseases including gestational diabetes in pregnancy, Type 2 diabetes, and cancer. Dr. Tobias's research has been published in leading scientific journals including the New England Journal of Medicine, and she has been recognized by the American Heart Association and the Society for Epidemiologic Research.

Top quote

"Rather than macronutrient compositions being incorrect or ineffective, I think it's the focus away from specific foods that is ineffective. For example, a low-carb diet can be comprised of healthy or unhealthy foods and the same is true with low-fat."

Is the vegan diet equally good for everyone?

"Vegan" refers to what is eliminated in the diet (animal products), but what is retained in that diet can span quite a large range of what is healthy or unhealthy. It's hard to say without knowing what is in the vegan diet.

What are the top risks of a vegan diet that you've seen, and how would you recommend avoiding those risks?

Building on the reply above, many foods are technically vegan but unhealthful. Simply avoiding animal products does not redeem the quality of refined carbohydrates, added sugars, and processed foods. There are concerns about B12 deficiencies, but I do not know the prevalence of that among vegan populations.

Three big meals or seven small meals?

Total calories and diet quality trump meal frequency or pace.

What purchase of fifty dollars or less has improved your ability the most to lead a healthy diet?

A weekly trip down the produce aisle and what ends up in my house has the biggest impact on what I eat.

What are the two foods you'd recommend that people should stop eating or drastically cut out?

The evidence against a place for red and processed meats in a healthful diet has accumulated substantially, and revelations for its environmental impact are the tipping point. They can and should be eliminated or drastically reduced in the diet.

What is worst advice you hear people give routinely in the nutrition community?

Focusing on a single food or nutrient can be misleading and provide a false sense of security that, "well, I'm avoiding this, so everything else must be okay." We don't consume nutrients in isolation. Nutrients make up foods and foods make up meals. This is why I believe putting dietary advice in the context of overall dietary and lifestyle patterns can be the most effective approach.

What's the top supplement or superfood that you recommend for everyone?

I am not sure that there is one.

Low-fat vs. low-carb diet for weight loss?

See my Lancet Diabetes and Endocrinology meta-analysis. The majority of the literature on low-fat are flawed trial study designs and, for the rest, it appears that low-carb is modestly better for long-term weight loss than low-fat.

However, as stated, interventions based on achieving a certain distribution of macronutrients have yet to consistently demonstrate effective long-term weight loss, even across a wide range of distributions (meaning very low-carb being better than very low-fat or vice versa).

Rather than the macronutrient compositions being incorrect or ineffective, I think it's the focus away from specific foods that is ineffective. For example, a low-carb diet can be comprised of healthy or unhealthy foods, same with low-fat. The focus on fat and carbs doesn't describe what actual foods should be consumed and it is open to gross misinterpretation and manipulation.

We still need to identify a dietary intervention that effectively leads to weight loss that is generalizable to a large population, and compliance will likely be the cornerstone to its success.

In the past few years, what attitude or belief has shaped your understanding the most about healthy nutrition and a healthy lifestyle?

The dietary pattern revolution has been a good model for nutrition epidemiologic research.

Population health in its current context of chronic diseases is unlikely to come down to a single dietary culprit. We've moved away from investigating the impact of single micronutrients, and are (slowly) coming around to realizing the unimportance of carbs vs. fat. Even the conversation of fats vs. carbs tends to quickly evolve into a discussion of healthful whole foods. As such, nutrition epidemiology is increasingly investigating overall diet, or dietary patterns, accounting for diet quality and the foods themselves.

Uncovering and quantifying the environmental impact of diet has also been really moving.

What do you do when you're craving junk food?

I don't really crave junk food. I do crave really good Mediterranean food that is sometimes difficult or time consuming to cook myself, so, I will get take-out, which is kind of a splurge.

Ekaterina Maslova

Dr. Ekaterina Maslova works as a Senior Epidemiologist at ICON Clinical Research. She also contributes to postgraduate teaching and student mentoring at the School of Public Health, Imperial College London. Dr. Maslova trained in nutrition and epidemiology at the Harvard School of Public Health and she did a postdoctoral fellowship at Statens Serum Institut, Danish Ministry of Health, examining the relationship between the nutrition during pregnancy of mothers with gestational diabetes and their children's health. She has published extensively in the field of pregnancy nutrition and child health and she serves as an Academic Editor for the journal, Nutrients. Dr. Maslova's research has contributed to the dietary recommendations for pregnant women in the USA and Europe.

Top Quote

"A vegan diet can be part of a healthy lifestyle for many, but it is not equally good for all. That is based on current evidence, but also on the common expectation that nutritional needs are different across a person's lifespan."

What book about nutrition do you frequently recommend to friends?

Eat, Drink, and Be Healthy by Prof Walter Willett and *Fast-Food Nation* by Eric Schlosser. I recommend the Willett book because it is a nutritional science book written for the general public which breaks down what we know and don't know about diet and health. It also does a good job of organizing evidence and tackling misconceptions about nutrition. The second book pushes the boundaries of what food is and discusses its evolution, attempting to make us pay closer attention to what we eat.

Is the vegan diet equally good for everyone?

A vegan diet can be part of a healthy lifestyle for many, but it is not equally good for all. This is based on current evidence, but also on the common expectation that nutritional needs are different across a person's lifespan. For example, fish intake in pregnancy and during breastfeeding has been shown to be beneficial for a range of maternal and child outcomes. For instance, fish is beneficial for allergic and metabolic diseases. An argument could be made that this benefit is due to Omega-3 fatty acids, which are also found in plant sources like nuts and seeds. However, the scientific evidence is strongest for studies that have examined fish intake and weaker for studies where scientists have measured only Omega-3 fatty acids intake or Omega-3 blood levels in participants. This seems to suggest that the entire food (the interaction among nutrients in fish) is important. Another example is that small children, because of their rapid growth, may benefit from Omega-3 fatty acids found in fish which do not need to be metabolized (can be directly used by cells) as opposed to Omega-3 fatty acids from vegetable sources, which need to be metabolized first.

What are the top risks of a vegan diet that you've seen, and how would you recommend avoiding those risks?

The biggest risk is probably not fully understanding the limitations of a vegan diet (for example, in terms of iron and B12 intake) and how to mitigate them through careful dietary choices. This also entails having a basic understanding of how certain combinations of foods are better than others. For example, eating green leafy vegetables with lemon juice or red peppers in order to optimize iron absorption, or avoiding tea with meals as it interferes with iron absorption. Unfortunately, the internet is brimming with unsubstantiated claims and urban legends when it comes to nutrition and people don't always have the time or energy to verify each claim. My recommendation is to look for references to peer-reviewed studies. Someone that cannot support their claims in a balanced manner (without cherry-picking articles) should inspire less trust than an author who carefully explains the evidence with all its limitations.

Three big meals or seven small meals?

The science is not clear on this question. There are some interesting studies in animals on caloric restriction and longevity and, more recently, data on intermittent fasting which in principle would favor fewer meals. However, how sustainable these are in humans under real life conditions is questionable. Past trials on caloric restriction have shown that, even with extensive support from nutrition professionals, caloric restriction is difficult to maintain. There are also good arguments for several meals per day; for example, that they could maintain blood sugar levels. While it might be disappointing that clear guidance doesn't exist on this issue, even if we had solid biological evidence, meal time and frequency (similarly to types of diets) are heavily guided by social and cultural factors which can make recommendations difficult to follow. Therefore, the regimen to adopt is the one that suits your lifestyle and allows you to eat a healthy and balanced diet.

What purchase of fifty dollars or less has improved your ability to lead a healthy diet the most?

Good glass containers that don't leech chemical coatings into the food, like perfluorinated compounds used for plasticware. Most people are familiar with BPA, but there are further substances in plasticware to avoid, and probably others that we are still unaware of or which haven't been tested in human studies. These substances are fat soluble and are therefore metabolized very slowly, meaning they can stay in your body for an extended amount of time. They are also not peaceful visitors and can interfere with your hormonal system (your long-distance signaling system) which can have adverse effects on health. This is truer for the unborn, infants, and children whose bodies are smaller but whose development is very fast (and, hence, very reliant on that long-distance signaling system).

What are the two foods you'd recommend to stop eating or drastically cut out?

A vegan diet is already good in avoiding some foods that contain carcinogenic substances and hormones that increase the risk for poor health outcomes (like red and processed meat, and dairy). Others, like sugar (including boiled potatoes and white bread), are well known. The ones that may be less known and less monitored by people are partially hydrogenated fat and coconut butter.

Partially hydrogenated fats, aka trans fats, is one food to stay away from. A man-made product, it has no benefits for your health and increases your risk of heart disease and diabetes. While many countries and US states have taken measures to ban trans fats from their food supply, most countries either haven't instituted measures or have partial measures in place, like voluntary reductions by industry and labels. With increasing public awareness, there is more pressure on industry to make changes, but there are no guarantees in countries where there is no ban. The next option would be to read labels. This is not always straightforward, and companies will try to deceive consumers by reporting the proportion of trans fat in a very small portion size, which can be misleading. Generally, no amount of trans fat is safe for consumption, so avoiding anything that has trans fat or partially hydrogenated fat on the label is the sensible approach.

The popularity of coconut oil has exploded in recent years, including in vegan cooking and baking. However, a lot of the health claims made about coconut oil are based on cell, animal, and small human studies, and often using pure ingredients from coconut oil rather than the oil itself. The majority of fat in coconut oil is saturated fat, most of which has been shown to raise 'bad' cholesterol. Medium-chain fatty acids, to which a lot of the health benefit of coconut oil is attributed, makes up only a fraction of these fatty acids. Virgin coconut oil does contain polyphenols, compounds that have important antioxidant properties, in amounts that are higher or similar to other polyphenols-rich foods like extra virgin olive oil and cocoa. These antioxidants may have some health benefits, but the evidence is still scarce. In the meanwhile, it is safer to limit consumption of coconut oil and turn to other liquid vegetable fats (like olive oil, rapeseed oil) where possible.

One supplement I recommend is vitamin D oil drops, especially if you live in the Northern hemisphere, apply sunscreen, or wear covering clothing. Since there are few good dietary sources for vitamin D, particularly if you don't eat animal products, taking some vitamin D oil drops can serve as an immune boost. This can help avoid colds or fight them during winter months. There is some data that vitamin D may also reduce the risk of chronic diseases like diabetes, some cancers, and heart disease. There is controversy regarding dosing as current recommended levels are based on skeletal outcomes and are quite low. Sun exposure to the face, neck, and arms for just a few minutes generates about 1,000 international units (IU) of vitamin D in the blood, but current recommendations are 200–400 IU per day. It is probably safe for an adult to take 5,000–10,000 IU if you don't get too much sun exposure or during cold/flu season. This is if you don't have any underlying conditions, in which case it is always advisable to consult your doctor.

Vitamin D is important during all stages of life, including pregnancy and breastfeeding (periods when the fetus is dependent on the mother for vitamin D) and infancy. Trials in pregnant women have given doses of up to 4000 IU without significant side effects. Young children require lower levels of vitamin D as significant side effects have been reported for children who have accidentally taken excessive vitamin D, but levels in children are much less studied. Recommendations vary between 400 and 1000 IU for children under 5 years. It is safest to give a breastfed infant or child (carried to term, without serious complications) vitamin supplements after they are six months old alongside vitamin D-rich or fortified foods. Baby formula is usually fortified with vitamin D and this should be considered when deciding whether to add additional supplements to a baby's diet. A popular urban legend is that high vitamin C helps during the cold/flu season. Trial data has shown that to not be the case. Vitamin C is a water-soluble vitamin so additional amounts that you consume are going to end up in your urine. Vitamin D is fat-soluble and stays in your system longer.

What is the worst advice you hear people give routinely in the nutrition community?

There is quite a lot of focus on protein intake in the general nutrition community. Yes, protein is important for proper physiological functions (as are carbs, fat, and micronutrients), especially among those that are very physically active or are professional athletes. However, the amount of protein we need is often exaggerated. Too much protein can, in fact, be bad for your health. There is evidence suggesting that too much protein can lead to poorer bone health (by increasing levels of acidity, leading to breakdown of bone), but also chronic conditions, like heart disease.

In studies of pregnant women, a higher protein intake has been shown to increase the risk of excess adiposity in their children later in life. Similarly, infants and children eating more protein have a higher risk of being overweight than children eating less protein. Like most things related to nutrition, moderation is key. Another thing to keep in mind is that protein sources are not created equal. Protein from vegetable sources have been shown to reduce risk of chronic disease like diabetes, while animal sources may increase these risks. The downside is that vegetable sources do not have a complete set of essential amino acids, so eating protein from a variety of sources (like legumes, nuts, seeds, grains, soy) is a good approach.

Low-fat vs. low-carb diet for weight loss?

Low-carb diets have strong biological arguments that favor them when it comes to weight loss. However, a few years back there was a study that looked at diets, including Ornish (low-fat) and Atkins (low-carb), and how they perform in terms of long-term sustainable weight loss. Although the low-carb diets performed better initially, in the long-term all diets actually performed similarly. Interestingly, the study found that the greatest weight loss was achieved by participants who could adhere to their diet, regardless of which type it was. So, the lesson is, if you want to lose weight, choose something that you can stick to.

Breakfast or no breakfast?

Definitely breakfast. Skipping breakfast is more likely to make you overeat later in the day and into the night. It is better to have a smaller dinner or an early one, and not go to bed on a full stomach and digest when the metabolism is working slower during the night. There is something to the saying, "Eat breakfast like a king and dinner like a peasant" (no disrespect to peasants or kings).

In the past few years, what attitude or belief has most shaped your understanding of healthy nutrition and and a healthy lifestyle?

In my research community (which studies nutrition in pregnancy and its influence on child health), the belief has long been that pregnancy is a crucial period for the future health of the child (which it is!) and that healthcare professionals should focus on changing the dietary habits of pregnant women. The assumption has been that pregnant women are more susceptible to change, but this has not been backed by data (apart from things like alcohol and caffeine). I think that actually makes a lot of sense.

Who would want to make drastic alterations to their diet when they're already dealing with big changes to their body and life in general? What has come out of this shift in belief is that, if diet needs to change, it needs to do so before pregnancy. There are also quite interesting evolutionary arguments supporting this, but it's somewhat outside the scope of this question. What is now an area of interest is when we should intervene in women's and men's lives to optimize health during pregnancy. I have an inkling that it will start moving down age groups to periods when dietary habits are established or susceptible to change, like childhood and adolescence. This will add another dimension to the role of nurseries, day care, and schools as they are some of the most influential institutions when it comes to improving public health.

What do you do when you're craving junk food?

Eat it. I find that trying to repress the craving just makes it worse. I usually eat enough to not crave it for a while.

Enette Larson-Meyer

D r. Enette Larson-Meyer is a registered dietitian and exercise physiologist who currently teaches and conducts research at the University of Wyoming. Her research interests focus on how nutrition influences the health and performance of active individuals at all stages of the lifecycle and at all levels of performance—from the casual exerciser to the elite athlete. Most recently, Dr. Larson-Meyer has become interested in vitamin D and iodine and the potential for these nutrients to influence the health and performance of athletes. Dr. Larson-Meyer is the author of *Vegetarian Sports Nutrition: Food choices and Eating Plans for Fitness and Performance* (Human Kinetics, 2007), is a former sports nutritionist for the University of Alabama at Birmingham, and served on the 2011 International Olympic Committee (IOC) Sports Nutrition Consensus Panel.

Top Quote

"We actually would have a bigger impact on human and environmental health if we got most of the population to become plant based vs. converting 1–2 percent of the population to be strict vegetarians."

What book about nutrition do you frequently recommend to friends?

It depends on the situation. I still like the Dean Ornish reversing heart disease books. I like the 100-mile diet to increase awareness of local foods and globalization, but I often recommend my own book to athletes and active individuals.

Is the vegan diet equally good for everyone?

Individuals following a vegan diet can meet all of their nutrient needs through selection of a variety of foods except for B-12 and iodine (if they do not use iodized salt). Some individuals are able to do this but, for others, a plant-based diet that contains a little dairy, eggs, or even fish, or sustainably-raised meat, is easier to follow. Also, if we are looking at environmental sustainability, many people who begin a vegan diet eventually quit following it because of their need to feel that one needs to be pure. We actually would have a bigger impact on human and environmental health if we got most of the population to become plant based vs. converting 1–2 percent of the population to be strict vegetarians. If you look at Joel Salatin's model of sustainable farming, animals such as chickens play an important role in the agriculture system that allows us to grow more healthy vegetables.

What are the top risks of a vegan diet that you've seen, and how would you recommend avoiding those risks?

First, people not being prepared for what they will eat. Second, not including a source of vitamin B-12. Third, the need to be pure. For example, vegans will be more successful if they ease into it and learn to cook more plant-based meals without meat, dairy, and eggs and also determine the strategies for what they will eat at restaurants, while traveling, etc. Vegans cannot live by salad alone. Learning to incorporate legumes, tofu, nuts, and seeds is key to meeting overall nutrient needs.

Three big meals or seven small meals?

I think it depends on lifestyle and energy needs. Some people like to snack. I advise my athletes with high energy needs to snack but it may be five or six small meals. I don't think this argument is particularly important.

What purchase of fifty dollars or less has improved your ability to lead a healthy diet the most?

Honestly, purchasing some kitchen "gadgets" that will whip up healthier meals and snacks. Some suggestions include: versatile serrated knife, quality apple slicer, quality egg cutter (also does mushrooms and strawberries), a small food processer, a basic crock pot.

What are the two foods you'd recommend to stop eating or drastically cut out?

My approach is to eat a balanced diet with a variety of healthy grains (whole and minimally processed), fruit, vegetables, nuts, seeds, legumes including tofu and, if desired, small amounts of cheese, yogurt, and eggs to accent flavors of food. Overall, I believe the healthiest diet is the Mediterranean diet that can easily be vegan or vegetarian.

What is the worst advice you hear people give routinely in the nutrition community?

Avoid carbohydrate or gluten as it makes you fat. Overeating anything makes people gain weight. Most foods people overeat are foods that contain both fat and carbohydrate (i.e., chips, donuts, fast food).

Low-fat vs. low-carb diet for weight loss?

Fat is important in our diets and helps enhance the flavor of our food. Carbohydrates are the preferred fuel of muscles during intense exercise and an important macronutrient. Both low-carbohydrate and extremely low-fat diets are not meant to be the way we eat. I believe in a balance like that recommended on the Mediterranean diet. With that said, however, carbohydrates should be from whole and minimally processed foods and fat choices should be from nuts, seeds, avocados, olives, and grapeseed oils that have a healthy fatty acid profile (lower in saturated and Omega-6 fatty acids).

Breakfast or no breakfast?

Breakfast is an important meal for many people but not everyone enjoys breakfast.

In the past few years, what attitude or belief has most shaped your understanding of healthy nutrition and a healthy lifestyle?

Studying nutrition and understanding the research and the benefit and function of healthy food has most shaped me. About ten years back, I realized that the food plate or food pyramid models of healthy eating (substituting protein food for meat) is ingenious. Each "food group" tends to be rich in certain nutrients and, if we strive to eat a variety of foods from each group, it is hard not to meet our nutrient needs.

What do you do when you're craving junk food?

I rarely crave junk food but, if I were, I would likely have it. I find if I am craving something, when I taste it, it does not taste as good as the craving would suggest. I feel our bodies figure out that this is not so good, either because the taste is not as good as we imagine or that we feel sort of sick after eating it. If we decide not to try it because we have too many food rules, then we can be ridden with guilt and this can lead to overindulgence later. Now, if I craved junk food daily, I would be answering this question differently. I would think that the junk food was making up for something else lacking in my life.

T. Colin Campbell

Dr. Campbell has been at the forefront of nutrition education and research for decades. Dr. Campbell's expertise and scientific interests encompass relationships between diet and disease, particularly the causation of cancer. His legacy, the China Project, is one of the most comprehensive studies of health and nutrition ever conducted. The New York Times recognized the study as the "Grand Prix of epidemiology." Dr. Campbell is the coauthor of the bestselling book, *The China Study: Startling Implications for Diet, Weight Loss, and Long-term Health*, and he is the author of the New York Times bestsellers, *Whole*: *Rethinking the Science of Nutrition* and *The Low-Carb Fraud*. He is featured in several documentaries including the blockbusters, Forks Over Knives, Eating You Alive, Food Matters, Plant Pure Nation, and others. He is the founder of the T. Colin Campbell Center for Nutrition Studies and the online Plant-Based Nutrition Certificate in partnership with eCornell.

Top quote

"Far too often, we seek truths and solutions that are so narrow in scope that they create really big mistakes."

What book about nutrition do you frequently recommend to friends?

I know this sounds ridiculously arrogant, but no book is devoted to nutrition with a wholistic interpretation. The discipline of nutrition science is so committed to reductionism that I cannot honestly recommend any book, except for those that give a good grounding in the chemical and physiological fundamental properties of nutrients and nutrient-like chemicals in food.

I spent my entire professional career teaching (introductory and upper-class teaching at university), conducting experimental research (with a multitude of students), developing national food and health policy (on expert committees with colleagues), and public lecturing (63 years), much of it in the usual reductionist mode. I have now sharply departed from that philosophy and can honestly say that the present science is bereft of that persuasion.

Is the vegan diet equally good for everyone?

I must add this background to answer your question. I don't use the word 'vegan.' In the biggest survey of its kind (the EPIC study in Europe), the average content of fat and sugar in vegan, vegetarian, and meat diets is exactly the same. Veganism and vegetarianism practices are mostly begun on ethical grounds, for good reasons, but I began my own journey in experimental research (in my graduate research program sixty-three years ago) from an opposite persuasion, high protein (animal protein) nutrition.

I came to my present views as a result of following the rules of science as faithfully as I knew how. That included publishing my work in professional peer-reviewed journals (about 350) while obtaining all of my relatively generous research funding (every last cent) from the public taxpayer (mostly NIH). It also meant that I sought critiques from audiences that were totally opposed to my interpretation of our research results (livestock enthusiasts, BIG PHARMA execs, geneticists). From that perspective, I called our evidence a whole food, plant-based diet (WFPB), a term (admittedly awkward) that I originated when I was first called on to describe it to a research grants advisory group of NIH, of which I was a member (about 1980). I did not want to call it vegetarian (I did not know the vegan word at that time) because it would have been a non-starter in a professional science community.

In answer to your question, therefore, I prefer to suggest my views of a WFPB diet as a goal. I prefer not proselytizing people to my point of view, as I value each person making their own choice. I believe my purpose, as a scientist, is merely to provide the best scientific evidence (especially because it was the public taxpayer who made my research work possible), then let others decide what to do with it. I believe that the closer one gets to a 100 percent WFPB diet, the healthier they will be, best shown when people with illness use this dietary lifestyle to treat and reverse their illness.

Yes, I have found that almost everyone (99 percent?) gains from this dietary lifestyle.

What are the top risks of a vegan diet that you've seen, and how would you recommend avoiding those risks?

I do not know of any significant risks, except perhaps the scorn people may get when choosing this option. Personally, I am at high risk for cardiovascular disease in my family while my wife (of fifty-six years) is from a family at risk for cancer. Thus, we gradually changed our diets as I began to acquire more and more convincing scientific information, obviously choosing this way of eating for ourselves and our immediate family—thanks to the brilliant development of tasty meals made by my wife.

I am eighty-five and take no drugs, while my wife at seventy-eight does the same. Also, our twenty-two-member family (children, grandchildren, spouses) do the same thing, with only one or perhaps two having slightly strayed on a few earlier occasions.

Three big meals or seven small meals?

Eat when you are truly hungry, but we follow the conventional three meals per day regimen.

What purchase of fifty dollars or less has improved your ability to have a healthy diet the most?

Will power—it is free. We don't use gimmicks (I don't mean to disparage others who do!). Sticking to an exercise routine is, of course, greatly helpful but we don't obsess about it.

What are the two foods you'd recommend to stop eating or drastically cut out?

I don't have a preferred answer. Perhaps, for myself, it was cheese. Once we are fully committed to this dietary lifestyle, it is easy. But this does require a commitment for at least 1–2 months for many people, a time during which we are clearing ourselves of our food addictions—especially those due to added oils, sugars, and fat.

What is worst advice you hear people give routinely in the nutrition community routinely?

I am presently writing another book and have devoted a full and lengthy chapter to this topic. I prefer to save this because it requires a longer discussion than is possible here.

Low-fat vs. low-carb diet for weight loss?

Read my book *Low Carb Fraud* (2016). Both the low fat and low carb concepts are poorly described, intended to gather attention, mostly for fame and fortune, and both lack scientific credibility. I would add one suggestion. Keep in mind that added oil and whole plant foods high in fat/oil are entirely different in their nutritional value, or lack thereof.

Breakfast or no breakfast?

Personal matter. Do what works best for yourself. I prefer a small breakfast because a big breakfast generates more hunger for the rest of the day.

In the past few years, what attitude or belief has most shaped your understanding of healthy nutrition and a healthy lifestyle?

It is the misconstrued concept in science—and, subconsciously, in everyday life—that is called reductionism. Far too often, we seek truths and solutions that are so narrow in scope that they create really big mistakes.

P.K. Newby

Dr. Newby is an Adjunct Associate Professor at Harvard, where she is an award-winning educator. She is a nutrition scientist and gastronome whose multidisciplinary training spans the biological, social, and public health sciences. Her mission is to help people live their healthiest, most delicious lives. She is a thought leader who speaks locally, nationally, and internationally, and her newest book is *Food and Nutrition: What Everyone Needs to Know* (Oxford University Press, 2018). Other works include "Superfoods" (National Geographic, 2016), and "Foods for Health: Choose and Use the Very Best Foods for Your Family and Our Planet" (National Geographic, 2014; with Barton Seaver). The responses below are excerpts from her book, *Food and Nutrition: What Everyone Needs to Know.*

Top Quote

"Nutrients lost in canning or freezing is not significantly different from fresh produce that is not consumed immediately and which begins losing nutrients once picked, so fresh or canned or frozen vegetables are all nutritious!"

What popular diets are best for weight loss?

Fad and celebrity diets and legitimate commercial weight loss plans have always been around to provide eaters with dieting options and each is touted as "the best." But is there really only one way to lose weight? Is one program truly superior? The basis for the efficiency of popular weight loss diets harkens back to biochemistry, e.g., the different effects of fat, carbs, and protein on appetite, food intake, and energy expenditure are key. Diets also differ not just in their composition but in other factors, too, including such things as social support, portion control, and food provision.

While many individual studies evoke provocative headlines, an example of a "single-study sensationalism," many are biased due to inadequate follow-up. Short-term weight loss is often different compared to results obtained over one year or more. A 2015 Cochrane review comparing Weight Watchers, Jenny Craig, Nutrisystem, MediFast, Opti-fast, Atkins, and SlimFast, for example, found that weight loss differences initially observed dissipated over a longer follow-up. Similar findings were seen in a rigorous review of Atkins, South Beach, Weight Watchers, and Zone diets, showing that all participants lost weight. And yet another meta-analysis found similar results comparing a wide range of popular low-fast and low-carb diets.

What does this all mean? Having some kind of plan is important, and following one that works for you is critical. Study after study shows that adherence is what leads to weight loss, not the diet particularly. (A clever nutrition professor made this point by following the "Twinkie Diet" losing twenty-seven pounds in ten weeks—though, to be clear, he also ate Oreos, Doritos, and powdered donuts. That said, don't do that!)

Do red and processed meats cause cancer?

While definitions vary, the WHO defines red meat as "all mammalian muscle meat including beef, veal, pork, lamb, mutton, horse, and goat." (No, pork is not "the other white meat," as US producers tout.) Processed meats begin with the base animal, usually pork or beef, and utilize salting, smoking, fermentation, and curing to enhance flavor and improve preservation or both. Common examples range from deli meats (e.g., ham, turkey, pastrami, bologna, salami) to fast food (e.g., chicken nuggets, hot dogs, pepperoni). Processed meats often hide in meat-based dishes and sauces, too.

While processed meats are generally higher in salt, sugar, and preservatives than unprocessed meats, both are sources of saturated fat and heme iron. Some processing methods involve nitrates, which are metabolized into N-nitroso compounds in the body—and the same compounds are produced in the gut following red meat consumption. Smoked meats can lead to the formation of polycyclic aromatic hydrocarbons (PAHs), as can cooking red meat at high temperatures, like grilling. The latter method also produces heterocyclic amines (HCAs). N-nitroso compounds, PAHs, and HCAs have all been shown to be cancer promoting agents in numerous lab and animal studies, spurring human studies examining red and processed meats. And heme iron, the kind found predominantly in meat, has been found to enhance HCA production through its metabolism which may lead to DNA mutations in the colon.

In 2014, the International Agency for the Research of Cancer convened twenty-two experts from ten countries to review more than 800 studies on RPM and cancer. The group concluded that processed meat was a group one agent (like tobacco) and carcinogenic. Specifically, 50 grams of processed meat consumed daily increases colorectal cancer risk by 18 percent. The evidence isn't as strong for red meat, with the IARC concluding it as "probably carcinogenic" in humans and that 100 grams of red meat consumed daily increases colorectal cancer risk by 17 percent.

Current studies are considering how the timing of intake across the life span, cooking method, and genetics impact the connection between RPM and colorectal cancer.

Are canned and frozen foods inferior to fresh?

Produce is usually processed at its peak and flash frozen at the same location where picked. This means maximal nutrients and vitamins are retained and maintained in your freezer. Thus, you can have even more vitamins and minerals compared to fresh produce that has been transported over a long period of time (particularly if conditions were suboptimal) or that sat around the market or house prior to consumption. Canning can lead to nutrient losses when vitamins leach into the liquid, just as when vegetables are boiled at home. But the amount lost is not significantly different from fresh produce that is not consumed immediately, and which begins losing nutrients once picked. (The vegetable is, after all, dying.) Yet some canned foods have even more nutrients than fresh as heating and cooking increase the bioavailability of some nutrients. For example, canned tomatoes—the most frequently consumed canned vegetable in the US—have a higher lycopene content than fresh, an antioxidant shown to reduce the risk of prostate cancer in many studies.

In summary, scientists actively study the bioavailability of specific nutrients across a wide range of foods, comparing fresh to frozen to canned—there are far too many exemplars to consider that vary across individual foods and the specific technology and storage conditions. The bottom line is that most people don't eat nearly enough vegetables and fruits for optimal health and disease prevention, and minimally processed foods help meet nutritional requirements (including canned and frozen foods).

Todd Binkley

Dr. Todd Binkley is a clinical nutritionist and chiropractor in Ventura, California. Dr. Binkley has practiced for over thirty years and has seen a wide range of nutritional and wellness issues.

Top Quote

"Even mild anemia, from B12 and/or iron deficiency, which most vegans I've tested have, puts a constant stress on the heart."

What book about nutrition do you frequently recommend to friends?

I usually recommend *Food Rules* (and anything else by Michael Pollan) and *Foods that Fight Cancer* by Denis Gingras and Richard Béliveau.

How much does diet really affect mood and psychological well-being?

Tremendously, in people with vitamin and mineral deficiencies, blood sugar issues, protein deficiency, and dysbiosis.

Is the vegan diet equally good for everyone?

It's theoretically fine for almost anyone, but functional protein, folate, B12, hydrochloric acid, and multiple mineral deficiencies are very common. Any vegan should get blood testing and nutritional analysis to confirm adequate absorption of these essential nutrients. Standard medical analysis of blood tests (which looks for the need for medical care, not for normal physiology) almost always misses these deficiencies. Even mild anemia, from B12 and/or iron deficiency, which most vegans I've tested have, puts a constant stress on the heart.

Three big meals or seven small meals?

The main reason to do several small meals is to reduce stress on the liver, and blood sugar spikes. For some, it's really important, for others it's not.

What purchase of fifty dollars or less has most improved your ability to have a healthy diet?

Vegetable seeds that I use to grow my own food, and show others how to do the same.

What are the two foods you'd recommend to stop eating or drastically cut out?

Soda, donuts, cupcakes, cookies, and fries.

What is the worst advice you hear people routinely give in the nutrition community?

Count calories and cut fat. That is unsustainable, because satiety is important. Learn how to make a delicious salad for four people, then eat the whole thing.

What's the top "superfood" or supplement that you recommend everyone should incorporate into their diet?

Vitamin D, 5000 IU daily for most adults.

Low-fat vs. low-carb diet for weight loss?

Low grains, low starch, and low sugar is better for most people. You can get all the carbs you need from spinach, broccoli, carrots, tomatoes, peppers, berries, and kale.

What is detoxification and how do you feel about the need for it?

I recommend against it without doing blood tests and nutritional analysis first. For many people, addressing unknown nutrient deficiencies is far more important. For some, stress on the liver, kidneys, and digestive tract need to be addressed first.

Breakfast or no breakfast?

Breakfast. The only good reason to skip it is to do intermittent fasting. Far better to skip dinner. You don't need food to sleep. The most important meal of the day for many people is lunch—

so that assimilated nutrients will be available to cells that night, when most healing and maintenance occurs.

In the past few years, what new attitude or belief has most shaped your understanding of healthy nutrition and a healthy lifestyle?

The benefits of intermittent fasting, and a ketogenic diet (about which there is much confusion).

What do you do when you're craving junk food?
Eat nuts, olives, and olive oil.

Janet Brill

Dr. Janet Brill is a nationally recognized expert in the field of health, wellness, and cardiovascular disease prevention and is frequently sought after by the media as a trusted source of nutrition and fitness information. She holds master's degrees in both nutrition and exercise physiology and a doctorate in exercise physiology. She is the author of three books: *Cholesterol Down, Prevent a Second Heart Attack,* and *Blood Pressure Down.* She has been published in noted scientific journals including the International Journal of Sport Nutrition, and the American Journal of Lifestyle Medicine.

Top quote

"Coffee is a definite. It's the main source of antioxidants in the American diet."

What book about nutrition do you frequently recommend to friends?

Cholesterol Down. It's my bestseller on lowering bad cholesterol with food and exercise. It's helped thousands of people around the world prevent cardiovascular disease and live a healthy lifestyle, without the risk of statin drugs.

Is the vegan diet equally good for everyone?

Theoretically yes, but practically I don't think so, as it takes a lot of planning and knowledge to eat a nutritious vegan diet. Many people do not have the desire to learn the correct way to eat vegan to ensure getting the nutrients required for good health.

What are the top risks of a vegan diet that you've seen, and how would you recommend avoiding those risks?

Building from the previous question, not eating enough (or not absorbing enough) of the top five are big risks. That's B12, Vitamin D, Omega-3 Fatty Acids, Zinc, and Iron.

Three big meals or seven small meals?

Whatever works for you, as long as the diet is nutritious and within the calorie range needed for a healthy weight.

What purchase of fifty dollars or less has improved your ability the most to lead a healthy diet?

I'll go with two: My Fitness Pal, a free food tracker app; and Stepz, a free walking tracker app.

What are the two foods you'd recommend to stop eating or drastically cut out?

First, red meat (associated with increased risk of disease and premature death).

Second, sweetened beverages (actually, if you cut out the liquid calories, you pretty much immediately slash the obesity epidemic).

On the flip side, if I had to recommend two foods, it'd be spinach and bananas. You can find them at every supermarket, they are inexpensive, sustainable, and highly nutritious. Regarding bananas, they are rich in potassium. Potassium is a mineral that Americans are not eating enough of. We eat a very high sodium and low potassium diet. This mineral imbalance contributes to the epidemic of high blood pressure (the silent killer) in this country.

What is worst advice you hear people give routinely in the nutrition community?

The irrational emphasis on the Paleo Diet. It's yet another fad diet high in animal protein and low in carbs! The best diet is a plant-based Mediterranean diet in my opinion.

Low-fat vs. low-carb diet for weight loss?

Definitely not low carb. I'd recommend a diet of moderate fat (extra virgin olive oil), whole grains, fruits, vegetables, nuts, and some Omega-3 rich fish. Basically, a normal healthy diet.

These days, there's a lot of talk about a low-carb diet lowering insulin levels, and therefore leading to fat loss. This is not the correct approach.

A healthy body releases insulin from the pancreas in response to glucose elevation in the blood. Insulin is the key that unlocks the door on the muscle cells allowing entry of glucose into the cells. Unhealthy Americans become insulin resistant meaning the insulin is less effective in unlocking the muscle "doors." Obese, inactive people tend to develop this situation, a precursor to type 2 diabetes. The best way to increase insulin sensitivity is to exercise and build muscle.

That said, insulin should not be the focus of weight loss. One of my favorite studies compared three diets for three months (high protein - low carb; low protein - high carb; moderate carb - moderate protein), and all were same caloric level. All three groups lost the exact same amount of weight. Eat less calories and burn off more through exercise is the age old formula for weight loss.

High protein diets make it easier to lose weight as protein is the most satiating macronutrient—the most filling. However, we as a nation eat far too much animal protein for good health. Adding vegetable protein to each meal and snack to fill you up (and eat a nutritious moderate carb and plant-based Mediterranean Diet) is a much healthier and satisfying strategy than the current high protein fad diets.

Breakfast or no breakfast?

Breakfast. Coffee is a definite (it's the main source of antioxidants in American diet). Coffee on an empty stomach isn't great, so something such as a banana if you can't fathom eating in the morning.

In the past few years, what attitude or belief has most shaped your understanding of healthy nutrition and a healthy lifestyle?

The Mediterranean Diet. It's a delicious plant-based eating style that's good for your health, the health of the animals, and the planet! Humankind must move to a plant-based green diet to sustain life on earth. This is quite profound, as our eating habits really do influence the future of this planet.

What do you do when you're craving junk food?

I eat it! However, not very often. The "secret" is that there is a plethora of healthy whole foods available that substitute for the junk-food craving. Dark chocolate, popcorn, etc., are healthy foods that cure the junk food cravings!

Joel Kahn

Dr. Kahn is the founder of the Kahn Center for Cardiac Longevity. He is a summa cum laude graduate of the University of Michigan School of Medicine and is a professor of medicine at Wayne State University School of Medicine. He is owner of Green Space Cafe in Ferndale, Michigan. His books, *The Whole Heart Solution*, *Dead Execs Don't Get Bonuses*, and *Vegan Sex*, all Number 1 best-sellers, are available for sale now. His public TV special, The Whole Heart Solution, is playing nationally now.

Top quote

Health is not an accident for most of us. It is a conscious decision to get to the gym or mat, to choose a side of greens over fries, to skip dessert or an entire meal, and to express gratitude daily.

What book about nutrition do you frequently recommend to friends?

In my medical practice, my special magic is referring patients to watch the smash video, Forks Over Knives, and then visit the website, forksoverknives.com. This documentary touches home on the message that food is medicine, that lifestyle is more important than genetics, and that reversal of chronic diseases can happen if you work at it. It is amazing, once you open the eyes of people to the possibility of healing, that they can control it and they can master it.

What are the top risks of a vegan diet that you've seen, and how would you recommend avoiding those risks?

There are three top dangers to veganism.

One is the trap of junk food. You can drink Mountain Dew and eat potato chips and not harm animals but you will harm your health. It has been shown by the Harvard School of Public Health and others that a plant diet of whole foods can lower the risk of heart disease but a junk food version can increase the risk. Beware.

The second danger is assuming a whole plant diet protects from all illnesses. This is simply not true. It may be the most powerful diet to prevent and reverse disease but most people have not done it for very long. I have eaten a whole food, plant only, diet for forty-two years and I still check my blood pressure, my lab studies, my colonoscopy, and other preventive measures.

Finally, the third pitfall is not supplementing. A whole food plant diet is better with B12, vitamin D3, and algae Omega-3. There are even some simple combination vitamins providing all three in one capsule or spray.

Three big meals or seven small meals?

Health is optimal with two meals a day and one midday snack. This is the recommendation of Valter Longo, Ph.D., author of *The Longevity Diet*, and the creator of the Fasting Mimicking Diet. That way you allow the body to heal and repair for at least twelve hours a day. Vitamin and antioxidant levels are replete. DNA is repaired. Injuries and stress from the daytime exposure to food and pollutants are renewed.

For most, eating is actually a necessary but disease-producing event that releases bacterial toxins into the bloodstream (metabolic endotoxemia). Eating plants wisely, and not too often, is the key.

What purchase of fifty dollars or less has improved your ability the most to lead a healthy diet?

A small blender (yes, some are under fifty dollars), allowing me to take 2–3 servings of greens, 2–3 servings of berries, ground flax seed, a plant milk, and spices and make an amazing morning drink. I do not blend it very much, as I like it chunky, and I actually chew it a bit to gain the advantage that eating and chewing green vegetables gives to healthy arteries. When green vegetables interact with bacteria on the tongue, it helps create nitric oxide for better arteries and blood pressure. If the smoothie is swallowed without any chewing, the greens may bypass the tongue and the full benefit is missed. Also, strong antiseptic mouthwashes can kill these friendly bacteria and should be avoided.

What is the worst advice you hear people give routinely in the nutrition community?

The worst advice is the ketogenic diet. This high-fat, low-carb, usually animal-rich diet may make you skinny for a while but serious studies involving over one million subjects raise the concern it may shorten your life. A bad tradeoff for a thinner waist for a while.

Low-fat vs. low-carb diet for weight loss?

Low fat is the key all the way. There are healthy diets moderately high in whole food sources of plant fats like nuts, olives, avocados, and maybe even olive oil, but these are higher in calories and some data still is of concern for plant oils and artery health. A whole food plant diet is low or modest in overall calories from fats and is optimal.

Breakfast or no breakfast?

Yes, the overall data is pro-breakfast. Some say, "eat breakfast like a king." But, after a minimum of a twelve hour break in eating (time-restricted feeding), I like oatmeal, berries, walnuts, and spices or a smoothie.

In the past few years, what attitude or belief has most shaped your understanding of healthy nutrition and a healthy lifestyle?

The risk to the environment has influenced my diet the most. We simply cannot feed the population and have a healthy planet if it is an animal food diet. Until factory manufactured animal foods are available, not involving an actual animal, we must stop eating animals. This is the message of the World Health Organization, the UN, the USDA, the EAT-Lancet panel, and others. When engineered animal foods arrive on the market soon, the decision to eat those products will no longer include animal slaughter and the degree of environmental destruction but, until then, it's clear what we should do.

What do you do when you're craving junk food?

When I crave food, I drink sparkling waters and grab a few frozen purple grapes. It totally satisfies the urges.

Heewon An

Heewon An is a clinical nutritionist in the Los Angeles area. She's been practicing nutrition for over fifteen years and has attended numerous seminars to broaden her insight, perspective, and knowledge about nutrition. She graduated from The University of Bridgeport with a Masters in Human Nutrition, while maintaining her role as a senior nutritionist at a nutrition and wellness clinic. In 2009 she started Healthee Life, a nutrition and wellness clinic in Los Angeles.

Top quote

"No one diet is good for everyone."

What book about nutrition do you frequently recommend to friends?

It really depends on what the friend or client needs. My clients typically want cookbooks or books on their condition. I haven't read any nutrition books recently but *Clean* by Dr. Junger was nice as I think most people can benefit from simplifying their diets and work on ridding toxins in their homes and environments. The *Encyclopedia of Natural Medicine* is another that I frequently looked to as a resource in my early learning days. Michael Pollan's books are great. I would recommend learning the why behind the "Whole 30" approach and my current interest, intermittent fasting. Nina Plank's books are good for those who need more of a foundational understanding of nutrition.

Is the vegan diet equally good for everyone?
No one diet is good for everyone. I've seen the vegan diet done well a few times and done poorly too many times. A vegan diet is difficult to do correctly because, by abstaining from all animal products, one needs to obtain all of his or her protein and vitamins from plants which can be difficult.

A purely vegan diet doesn't reflect any indigenous diets of the world as many seemingly vegan cultures actually used insects and such in their diets. That being said, the people of the blue zones eat very little meat, maybe a small portion 1–2 times a month. The blue zones are the mysterious regions where people statistically live the longest. They are: Sardinia, Italy; the islands of Okinawa, Japan; the Nicoya Peninsula in Costa Rica; Ikaria, Greece; and Loma Linda, California. The meat that is eaten may comprise of fish and the other muscle meats we are accustomed to but they generally include organ meats. Those peoples also eat mostly carbohydrates and very little fat.

A note about the blue zones of the world. They are relatively secluded, and unpolluted, and they still have a small network of people. Like a village, so to speak. Thus, the physical and emotional weight in these communities are very different from ours. We lack the type of small town social connection, we may live far away from family, and our bodies are bombarded with the stresses of modern life: chemical assaults and EMF, radiation, long work hours, etc. I mention this because, after twelve years of clinical practice, these toxins of modern life cause a lot of harm. To ward off the damage, the body requires enough nutrients, like protein and the B vitamins to support phase one and two liver detoxification.

We are living in a time when our grains are genetically modified, our meats and dairy are pasteurized and full of antibiotics and hormones, and our fruits and veggies have pesticide contamination. Each individual really needs to find what suits his or her genetic makeup AND his or her current environmental challenges and go from there. A new interest of mine is creating nutrition programs based on genetic malfunctions (genetic testing) as well as epigenetic ones.

What are the top risks of a vegan diet that you've seen and how would you recommend avoiding those risks?

I have clients and friends who are vegan for a variety of reasons but usually they are vegan because they don't want to eat animals—for spiritual reasons, animal rights, cultural, etc., AND/OR they don't feel good eating meat. If it is the latter, typically they aren't what I call the junk food vegetarians/vegan.

I really do want to educate people about moving away from factory farmed meats, so, really looking at why a whole food group is restricted would be a good start. It's hard when autoimmunity is on the rise and food sensitivities are growing (I think due to GMO's), so, I work with vegans who are sensitive to grains and beans and sometimes can't digest nuts. Soaking and sprouting these can aid digestion but I believe vegans need a good protein source (hemp is usually okay) and B vitamins (nutritional yeast) to start.

Three big meals or seven small meals?

Again, it depends. I've seen people succeed either way but snacking too often or eating too often can set you up for low blood-sugar-related symptoms. Our bodies are adaptable, so, if you start eating every two hours and then miss a snack, it will ASK for food. Also, the thing about snacks is that no matter how nutrient-dense the snack, they are typically not balanced. I'd rather people eat four meals instead of snacking on bars and random things throughout the day. Be intentional when eating. I am personally moving toward intermittent fasting but I don't think that's necessary for everyone. Some may not need this kind of time frame to eat enough or not overeat and some may possibly do damage because, like anything else, it needs to be done right. The most important thing is to eat enough of the right foods.

What purchase of fifty dollars or less has improved your ability the most to lead a healthy diet?

Lately, a free app, My Fitness Pal. I was against the notion of counting calories so had my clients use basic measuring comparison by hand. But actually, inputting everything I ate and seeing where each macronutrient tallied up was really insightful. Along with this, maybe a food scale would be useful.

The most important thing you cannot buy. It's mindset. Because we have to make food and lifestyle decisions all day long. Thus, planning is the key to good nutrition. Plan so you don't have to make a million decisions when you're hungry! I struggle with this all the time.

What are the two foods you'd recommend to stop eating or drastically cut out?

Food includes anything that comes out of the ground or from a living being in which case I wouldn't take out any one or two foods for everyone. We are all unique. I personally limit gluten-containing grains and dairy but you may be okay with good quality grains and raw dairy. I choose to avoid these, in addition to soy and sugar, because of the countless studies that point to these foods as being inflammatory. There are just too many success stories of beating autoimmune diseases after cutting out these foods. I've tested so many people in my office and these foods are generally not good for most. But, again, not everyone has the same sensitivities.

If we are talking about "food"—like anything we can buy at a store? I couldn't name just two.

I would have to say anything in a box.

Or anything with an unpronounceable ingredient in it.

Processed carbohydrates—cereals, breads, chips, crackers, the list goes on (these aren't real foods).

Rancid fats—bad oils—canola, margarine, soy oil, vegetable oil, and then anything fried in these bad oils—these cause the most damage, through oxidative stress.

And just for fun—chemicals, hormones, antibiotics, food colorings, artificial flavoring, etc.

Fortified foods—if it needed to be "healthified" with synthetic nutrients, it's probably highly processed.

What is the worst advice you hear people give routinely in the nutrition community?

Maybe not the worst, but the first one that comes to mind is a misconception that salt is bad for us. It is true that we as a modern species eat significantly too much processed salt (white table salt). Salt that is properly air dried, unrefined, and unbleached is essential for our digestion, immune function, and nervous system. I recommend pink salt from the Himalayas or from Hawaii (my choice). It's hard even with these pink salts to know if they are air dried (vs kiln dried).

Low-fat vs. low-carb diet for weight loss?

Neither is ideal. Both will work because most weight problems happen when we eat too much fat with too much carb (i.e., hamburgers, pizza, chocolate, etc.), so, the fat we eat gets stored. Naturally, carbs are our bodies' preferred source of fuel. So, to cut out all carbs isn't ideal for the body. The low fat diet crazes of the 1990s showed much evidence on the harm that can occur as we age without adequate fat. We need to be able to burn both, use both carbs and fat for fuel.

Many of us get stuck with fat loss resistance (I say fat loss, not weight loss) because of the cell receptor damages from either our genetics or environment or both (i.e., insulin receptors, leptin receptors, vitamin D receptors) that cause hormonal imbalances in the body. The fuel isn't the problem, it's that we've become too reliant on only being able to burn sugar. So, we go low carb and the body forgets how to burn sugar, so, it stores it once again as fat. We go low fat and then lose energy, get depressed, and our skin gets dry, etc. We need both. I'm not a fitness expert but many seem to settle somewhere around a 40–carb–30 fat–30 protein breakdown of where our calories should come from, basically balance.

I have been dabbling with carb cycling—alternating moderately high carbs and low carbs days—and I feel that this is the best option out there for fat loss and maintenance while getting in all the nutrients (fats and carbs) because restriction typically isn't sustainable.

Breakfast or no breakfast?

I was taught the importance of "eating within an hour of waking" long before I started studying nutrition, so, despite the many years of my teenage years that I didn't eat breakfast, I started eating earlier. And I did gain weight. I attributed it to just eating more, although not 100 percent sure. Other than the weight gain, I'm not sure if I noticed any big changes.

Last year, the myriad reports of people feeling better, getting rid of brain fog, and having more energy had me really curious about intermittent fasting. So, I started it almost a year ago and I am still doing it. For me, it's more the night time snacking that is a problem, so, intermittent fasting takes that away. I like that I look forward to eating and I appreciate my meals a lot more. It helps me to be mindful at mealtimes and discourages eating my toddler's leftovers for lunch and then, because of the calorie deficit, finding myself with the munchies at 9:00 p.m. So, breakfast or not isn't so much the question. I like how Dr. Masters calls it "concentrated meal times." You can have breakfast (as in eat in the morning), and stop eating earlier in the afternoon and still have the same results. Again, it depends on when wake time and bedtime is for each individual.

I've always suggested that people give the body at least four hours before bed to properly digest dinner, so, that could be a factor. One person I met wakes at 3:00 a.m., goes hiking, eats brunch around 7:00–9:00 a.m., then finishes dinner around 3:00–4:00 p.m. So, she is participating in an eight hour feeding window but has been doing this for thirty years. Even with all the hype on intermittent fasting these days, she probably doesn't realize that she's practicing anything other than what fits her lifestyle.

In the past few years, what attitude or belief has most shaped your understanding of healthy nutrition and a healthy lifestyle?

I've always believed in the limitless ability of the body to heal given the proper nutrients. However, that road isn't necessarily easy or simple. As I answered above, it's mindset first—attaining the deep understanding that we should eat to nourish our bodies (vs. eating for pleasure) and then find our why—to take care of our bodies because _______. (Fill in the blank: to be there for our grandkids, to have the energy to change the world in your own unique capacity, etc.)

What do you do when you're craving junk food?

Cravings aren't all bad but they can be difficult to decipher. If the craving is bigger than you (getting out of bed to sneak-eat a bowl, or the whole pint, of ice cream) it probably isn't our minds. There is something deeper, typically a complex village of bacteria, virus, and yeast inside of you that need to be fed. In this case, these underlying issues need to be addressed.

Sometimes, however, it's because our bodies need something that we didn't feed it. I wrote about my night time munchies. Generally, cravings happen when we are deficient. It could be a macronutrient or a micronutrient or both. Craving something salty? You are probably low in minerals. Craving sugar? Could be low in protein or just calories. Specific cravings tell us a lot about what the body needs. One of the most profound statements I heard while I was a student was that malnutrition is the beginning of obesity. We keep eating because our brain keeps telling us it needs something but we are feeding it junk, high calorie, low nutrient-dense "foods."

So, when I have a real craving, I try to ask myself what I really need. But it's a balance, and I like to have fun! And I have little kids! So I try to live by my recommendations to my clients and to make a place or time for that thing you really love and have it on Saturdays or Sundays. And FULLY enjoy it. Make it worth it. Don't regret it. At parties, I have something if I really want it. When traveling, I typically fast (I've incorporated 24–hour fasts weekly.) When I was in France, I ate dessert after every meal and drank coffee and felt great. Was it the vacation? The walking five or more miles everyday? The air? The quality of their wheat and milk? I don't know.

A practical thing I do each night is brush my teeth with my kids at 6:30 or 7:00 p.m. way before I myself am going to bed because I'm done eating. It's helped tremendously for sticking to abstaining from eating at night. My thing was ice cream. I could eat ice cream for dinner in college, if no one else was around and I was too busy to eat. As I got healthier, I wanted it less. And now, I don't want regular ice cream. I find way more satisfaction out of eating a coconut milk ice cream sweetened with wild honey. And when all I want to eat are crackers and noodles, I know something is up. It could be emotional or physical. Finding help is another way of taking responsibility for this crazy body of ours.

Kelsey McGuire

Kelsey is a nutritionist at the Chicago Department of Public Health. She supervises staff, assesses the nutritional needs of the population, and develops nutrition care plans. She oversees the Women Infant Children program. The WIPC is a federally funded program implemented by the City of Chicago that provides pregnant, breastfeeding, and postpartum women, and children and infants with nutrition assistance.

Top quote

"I believe in breakfast."

Is the vegan diet equally good for everyone?

No, everybody has different needs. Vegan diets often lack iron, and women of childbearing age have higher iron needs compared to men. Also, just because something is vegan does not make it healthy. Some people will make healthier food choices over others.

What are the top risks of a vegan diet that you've seen, and how would you recommend avoiding those risks?

Lack of nutrients. Cutting out food groups can lead to vitamin and mineral deficiencies especially. I would recommend eating complete proteins as much as possible, and consulting a medical doctor for lab work because these vitamin and mineral deficiencies are not obvious.

Three big meals or seven small meals?

It depends on the person and their day-to-day activities. Waiting too long between meals may lead to overeating if the person isn't eating slow enough or listening to their internal satiety cues. Grazing can work for some, but many people underestimate how many calories they are eating. A snack may actually turn into a small meal.

What purchase of fifty dollars or less has improved your ability the most to have a healthy diet?

Digital food scale. I'm able to portion foods, and it helps with cooking and baking measurements.

What are the two foods you'd recommend to stop eating or drastically cut out?

Soda, since there is zero nutritive value. Anything with trans fat because there are clear links to heart disease. I'd recommend any green leafy vegetable. Also, I don't really believe in the term, "superfood."

What is the worst advice you hear people give routinely in the nutrition community?

These days, you hear a lot about cutting out carbs completely. I believe all foods fit in a diet, and cutting out food groups may lead to deficiencies. People forget that carbs are in many foods and beverages. People need to evaluate which carbs are a better choice, and know that carbs are your bodies' preferred fuel.

Low-fat vs. low-carb diet for weight loss?

Low-carb is trending right now. I think portion control is more important, however. Choose unsaturated fats over trans and saturated fats. Choose whole grains, and complex carbs.

Breakfast or no breakfast?

I believe in breakfast. It sets the stage for your day, gives you an opportunity to fuel your morning, and gives you the energy to make healthy choices throughout the day.

In the past few years, what attitude or belief has most shaped your understanding of healthy nutrition and a healthy lifestyle?

There is no one size fits all approach. Nutrition and lifestyle choices need to be tailored to an individual, and those will change over time. Take small steps to get started and be realistic about maintenance.

What do you do when you're craving junk food?

I allow myself to partake in a treat occasionally. I just make sure to keep portions in check.

Brenda Davis

Brenda Davis, Registered Dietitian, is a leader in her field and an internationally acclaimed speaker. She has worked as a public health nutritionist, clinical nutrition specialist, nutrition consultant, and academic nutrition instructor. Brenda is the lead dietitian in a diabetes research project in the Marshall Islands. She is a featured speaker at nutrition, medical, and health conferences throughout the world.

Brenda is co-author of nine award-winning, best-selling books: *Becoming Vegan: Comprehensive Edition* (2014), *Becoming Vegan: Express Edition* (2013), *Becoming Vegan* (2000), *The New Becoming Vegetarian* (2003), *Becoming Vegetarian* (1994, 1995), *Becoming Raw* (2010), *The Raw Food Revolution Diet* (2008), *Defeating Diabetes* (2003) and *Dairy-free and Delicious* (2001). Her books are vegetarian and vegan nutrition classics with over 750,000 copies in print in eight languages.

Top quote:

"No diet is equally good for everyone. Every person has a unique metabolism."

What book about nutrition do you frequently recommend to friends?

I recommend the award-winning classics, *Becoming Vegan*, *Comprehensive or Express Edition.* They are the most detailed, reliable, evidence-based vegan nutrition guides available. These books cover diet and disease, macronutrients and micronutrients, guidelines for pregnancy, lactation, infancy, childhood, adolescence, seniors, athletes, underweight, overweight, eating disorders, and practical information including a food guide and menus.

Is the vegan diet equally good for everyone?

No diet is equally good for everyone. Every person has a unique metabolism and gut microbiome, so, there are numerous variables that will impact response to food. Some people have allergies and sensitivities to foods and, if they are sensitive to legumes, nuts, and seeds, eating 100 percent plant-based can be more challenging. However, a well-designed vegan diet will consistently reduce risk of chronic disease and, in many cases, effectively treat these diseases. For most individuals, meeting nutritional needs on a vegan diet is not difficult, providing the diet is well planned.

What are the top risks of a vegan diet that you've seen, and how would you recommend avoiding those risks?

The top risks are nutritional deficiencies such as vitamin B12, vitamin D, and iodine. These are easily avoidable with supplements or fortified foods. Some very restrictive vegan diets can be hazardous, especially for small children. Again, this is easily avoidable by including a wide variety of nutritious foods, and including sufficient legumes, including soy foods such as tofu and tempeh.

Three big meals or seven small meals?

I think this depends on the individual. For people who need fewer calories, or who are overweight, I think eating less often is preferable. For those who require a lot of calories (e.g., athletes), eating more often can be very helpful. Small children need to eat more often as well.

What purchase of fifty dollars or less has improved your ability to have a healthy diet the most?

No question, mason jars. They make it so easy to be organized and efficient in the kitchen, and they double as sprouting jars. I have about sixteen mason jars in the freezer part of my fridge (mainly for nuts and seeds), and at least as many in the pantry (for beans and grains). They are all clearly labeled and accessible.

What are the two foods you'd recommend to stop eating or drastically cut out?

I would say to stop eating highly refined carbohydrates, sugars and starches (sugar and flour products), and fried foods. Refined carbohydrate foods (like sweet beverages and all the white flour products—breads, crackers, cookies, etc.) increase the risk of diabetes, heart disease, and cancer. Fried foods, or foods containing a lot of added fat, are also highly damaging to health. Generally, you want to get carbohydrates from whole plant foods like vegetables, fruits, whole grains, and beans; and fats from whole plant foods like nuts, seeds, avocados, and organic soybeans. As for foods I highly recommend, my top five foods would be dark leafy greens, legumes (beans and lentils), Omega-3 rich seeds (flax, chia, hemp), berries, and vegetables of all colors.

What is worst advice you hear people give routinely in the nutrition community?

I would say it is to eat a high fat keto or paleo-style diet. These diets are very high in total and saturated fat, and can be low in protective dietary components like fiber, phytochemicals, and antioxidants—especially keto diets, which are nutritionally lacking. Paleo diets are very high in meat, which increases risk of cancer, diabetes, and heart disease, and they are unsustainable ecologically.

Low-fat vs. low-carb diet for weight loss?

In my opinion, the balance of macronutrients (protein, fat, and carbohydrate) is far less relevant than the sources of those macronutrients. When calories come from whole plant foods (vegetables, legumes, fruits, whole grains, nuts, and seeds), and energy balance is maintained, great health can be achieved with a range of macronutrient intakes. All of that having been said, low-carb means low plant, as all plant foods (with the exception of nuts and seeds) provide about 58–92 percent of calories from carbohydrate. So low-carb diets are generally low-plant diets. The lowest carb foods are meat, poultry, fish, and eggs.

Breakfast or no breakfast?

Breakfast for sure, although it depends somewhat on your body clock. I am a morning person, so, I am hungry within an hour or two of rising. I have no desire to eat after dinner as my body is winding down. Others, who are night people, may be the opposite. We do need to listen to our bodies. My general rule is eat when you are hungry and don't eat if you are not hungry. However, eating a nutritious breakfast provides energy and valuable nutrients to help get you through the day, so, it is generally advisable.

In the past few years, what attitude or belief has most shaped your understanding of healthy nutrition and a healthy lifestyle?

I would say the concept of getting our macro and micronutrients from whole foods rather than from highly processed foods. It is better to get carbohydrates from fruits, vegetables, beans, and grains than from sugars and starches that were extracted from those foods. It is better to get protein from beans, tofu, tempeh, nuts, and seeds than from proteins isolated from those foods. It is better to get fat from nuts, seeds, and avocados rather than the oils extracted from those foods. The reason is simple. When the macronutrients are extracted from their original whole foods, most of the protective factors like fiber, phytochemicals, and antioxidants are left behind during processing.

What do you do when you're craving junk food?

I don't crave "junk food." I crave salad, peaches, and blueberries! This happens when your palate adjusts to the amazing natural flavors of whole foods. When I feel like having a special treat, I go for stuffed dates or dark chocolate treats (homemade and stored in the freezer), ice cream (made from frozen bananas, mango, and pineapple), and, occasionally, popcorn.

Melissa Yee

Melissa began her career as a functional nutritionist after a debilitating eye disease and the side effects of antibiotic chemotherapy led her to the Nutritional Therapy Association. She enrolled in the Nutritional Therapy Practitioner program to direct her own healing process and quickly fell in love with the company and its mission to empower individuals, cultivate a community, and heal the world.

Melissa believes that true health is always bio-individual—an artful and dynamic blend of science, philosophy, and a lived experience. She is a Certified Nutritional Therapy Practitioner from the Nutritional Therapy Association.

Top quote

"Any kind of dogmatic diet doesn't honor the individual's bio-individuality."

Is the vegan diet equally good for everyone?

You really need to see a person in their philosophical framework and whether veganism is highly philosophical for them and, for some reason, the person doesn't want to eat meat. Animal parts, particularly fats, are some of the most bioavailable nutrition. Because the meat industry is so bad, and animal farming is so unhealthy, making a conscientious plant-based diet can be healthier than making the choice of poorly-sourced animal foods.

I don't think any one diet is good for anyone ever. Everything has to vary for the individual, not only genetics and epigenetics.

Microbiome is very important for what your current needs are. Just being frank, it's difficult to maintain optimal fat soluble vitamin balance (particularly A) and protein.

If you look at people like Rick Roll, you have a team of nutritionists tweaking their diets all the time. But it doesn't have to be black or white! Certain indigenous tribes that are known to be the most long-living, do consume animal products from time to time. It's also really important to optimize for protein. Chickpeas and lentils have protein, but your body doesn't recognize it the same way.

You can't ignore ancestry, where your people came from, and what the ancestral diet was. You can't be dogmatic about anything. When you're conscientious, intuitive, and smart enough to work with a functional medicine doctor to catch deficiencies early, you can make the diet that you want work. Nutrition is very personal. Anytime very strong and personal values come into play, it's very important to optimize within that framework. But you have to do it carefully and with responsibility, to avoid the mental biases that are associated with dogma, and make it work for you. You have to go about it in an educated way and continue monitoring.

What are the top risks of a vegan diet that you've seen, and how would you recommend avoiding those risks?

Vitamin A, D, E; fat soluble vitamins

What my clients came to me about symptomatically: fatigue, lethargy, bloating/some sort of stomach issues, acne/eczema.

The underlying root causes of all the above was poor fatty acid balance which contributed to poor absorption of fat-soluble vitamins. Protein balance was also an issue.

Fatty acid deficiency. There's a balance of fatty acids that we need: omega-3, 6, and 9 to make the body function properly. Omega-3 is anti inflammatory and omega-6 is inflammatory. When you see a client and they are presenting a lot of inflammatory immune symptoms, you can generally infer that the omega-6 balance is on the high side compared to omega-3 balance. The point is that the ratio is tricky to maintain as a vegan because it's not good to consume various synthetic oils (palm, canola, mixed vegetable oils). Iron deficiency is also very common. Fatty acid deficiency also relates to not being satiated after meals and high prediabetic blood sugar (even though many clients were young, not overweight).

The point is that so many of these issues that I saw were actually intertwined. For example, one of the risks was vitamin A. Even if you're getting a ton of beta-carotene, if you're not consuming enough of the right fats, it's just not getting absorbed. These risks are possible to avoid. It's possible to get enough of the nutrients, but you have to be very conscious and careful. If you're having nuts, they have to be thoroughly soaked. Also, you have to be mindful about vitamin intake and make sure you get high quality fats that allow you to absorb these foods.

Our bodies are made to digest fat and sometimes people tell me, "I can't eat fat." But really, they also have an enzymatic deficiency. In order to digest the foods in your stomach, you need to have sufficient enzymes and sufficient stomach acid. You have to break down the food, and also break down the pathogens that get into the stomach. Your stomach should be reaching a pH of 1–3. If you're not producing enough of these enzymes and acids, your body isn't in a relaxed state, and what happens is that the food isn't properly digested. It gets passed on without proper digestion. You can get an immune response and all sorts of digestive issues. You need to be in a relaxed state and then your brain will trigger all the autonomic functions that your body needs. Some people are unstoppable train engines who have adapted to high stress lifestyles. But, for the most of us, our stomachs won't produce adequate acid and our gallbladders won't produce adequate enzymes if we are in a neurotic state. You could eat the most perfect combinations of foods but, if you're a neurotic stress case, and you don't chew your food, and you eat while running from meeting to meeting, you can still be nutritionally deficient.

Another issue is orthorexia, an eating disorder where people are highly restrictive about their diet. Any community where people are obsessed about the food they eat (paleo, vegan, keto, etc.), it's not about the diet but the act of obsessing over the food itself that is very unhealthy because it doesn't allow your mind to be at peace and digest properly. You could even say that meditation is the most important vitamin—carving out the time to breathe a little bit before eating, look at the food, and let your body get into the proper state.

Three big meals or seven small meals?

That depends on your blood sugar status. It also depends on your overall digestive status. Typically, I prefer fewer large meals, because you give your digesting system time to rest. I highly recommend also prioritizing a twelve hour fast, because digesting takes a lot of energy away from other internal processes. If you're eating all the time, that is a problem because there are a lot of hormonal processes and endocrine functions that require you to not be digesting at all.

When you have a job that's around the clock, and your brain is awake, it's hard to not be hungry at night and to not eat. If your goals outweigh your considerations for health, that's a choice. If you really need something to sleep, a moderate well-balanced snack is good. But, ideally, not eating before you sleep is the best because a lot of neuroregenerative processes occur. If you do eat a snack at night, make sure that it's well balanced. Overall, having an eating schedule that's misaligned with your circadian rhythm is quite damaging.

Drinking coffee in the morning, instead of eating, depends on your particular status. If you feel like you're not depleted, have some with some fat. But if you have problems with your blood sugar, it's not a great idea. The reason it's better to have coffee with something is because it stimulates cortisol production and I know, anecdotally, that many of my clients don't do well on coffee on an empty stomach. It's better to have it with some fat or half an avocado or something. In general, coffee isn't great if you're suffering from adrenal dysfunction or blood sugar dysfunction.

If someone has severe hypoglycemia, many small meals could be appropriate. But I generally only recommend that as a temporary diet and it's important to get to a place where one can eat less frequently in order to allow the body to rest.

What purchase of fifty dollars or less has improved your ability to have a healthy diet the most?

Right now something I'm really loving is propolis and bee pollen.

What are the two foods you'd recommend to stop eating or drastically cut out?

For the general audience, it's generally sugar. For vegans, they typically care about their body, and I'm assuming they already cut out sugar and highly processed foods.

The other really important things are highly processed vegetable oils such as canola, hydrogenated oils, sunflower seed oil, and any processed oil because they are very high in omega-6 and small quantities of trans fats. I would replace them with olive oil, avocado oil, and coconut oil (especially for high heat). You can find cost-effective versions of these oils. If you can afford cold-pressed avocado oil, that's another great option.

I would recommend excluding gluten and seeing how one does. Not everyone is gluten intolerant but it can do a lot of damage and many people are gluten intolerant, so, it makes sense to avoid it.

Separately, cut out stress around eating! As I described in the previous questions, being relaxed and happy around eating, being hydrated, is the easiest change to make.

What is worst advice you hear people give routinely in the nutrition community?

Any advice that says, "you must have this diet" (insert paleo, keto, vegetarian, etc.) and anything dogmatic that doesn't honor bio-individuality. People shouldn't give answers without respecting the individual autonomy of the individual. Nothing will work for everyone.

A fruit juice fast is so horrible for people who have blood sugar issues. It can tip them over the scale to a prediabetic zone in a week. For women in particular. Also fasting, in general, for people who have diabetic issues.

Low-fat vs. low-carb diet for weight loss?
In general, I would recommend low carb. But it also depends. Many people can lose weight on a balanced diet. It takes investigation to understand why the person gained weight in the first place. If it's mental or emotional, than it's usually not the diet.

I've worked with so many people and, typically, people have tried the conventional things and they haven't worked. If I'm looking at someone who has no other factors, I would see what their diet was beforehand and, if they were eating a lot of carbs, I would transition them to a more low-carb diet. If they were eating a lot of fats, I would transition them to a more balanced fiber-rich diet. It's a tricky question without working one on one with people.

Breakfast or no breakfast?
The most important principle is making sure you have that twelve hour time between the meals, for reasons explained above. However, it really depends on the individual! Some people do well skipping breakfast. If you feel strong, energetic, and happy in the morning, then it's fine. I see skipping breakfast not working well, in particular, for women.

In the past few years, what attitude or belief has most shaped your understanding of healthy nutrition and a healthy lifestyle?
A really important concept is balancing intuition with observation. Einstein is one of my biggest influencers. He captured so many things beautifully and he understood that the scientific world is tied up in our spiritual beliefs.

In nutrition, the ability to live well is highly dependent on the ability to understand how you're doing. How is your sleep? How do you feel? Many people have lost the ability to know how they are feeling. But what we perceive as reality can be a deception. So, you have to balance that with observation (getting tested, looking at those numbers) and react appropriately.

Pay attention to how you're feeling. Keep a log! Tests should verify what you already feel. In a way, it's a scientific attitude. The intuition creates a hypothesis that you have, and you have to use observations to see if it's true or not and evolve from there. One thing that made a big difference for me was tracking when I felt tired or bloated. Seeing that "data" allowed me to see patterns of the kinds of things triggered those feelings.

What do you do when you're craving junk food?

I usually question why. Am I stressed and on a deadline? Am I looking for a diversion? If I'm craving something sweet or fatty, I'll try to make a healthy similar thing. For example a mocha latte with butter or cocoa milk, something that feels luxurious and healthy. But every now and then, I'll just do it! You have to question what life is about. It's not about your perfect diet! If you're making informed decisions, and doing it within reason, it's not going to kill you! Of course, if people have certain health conditions, that advice could change. You have to be reasonable.

Tessa Englund

Tessa received her Ph.D. in Nutrition from Virginia Tech, where she researched large-scale strategies to promote healthy and sustainable food environments and consumer behaviors. Tessa is passionate about the plant-based lifestyle, and has dedicated her career to promote a healthier environment and greater overall health in the human population.

Top Quote

"Diet has a strong relationship with mood, which is much more notable when acute nutritional needs are not met or are exceeded."

What book about nutrition do you frequently recommend to friends and clients?

Honestly, I don't have any one book that I can think of! I do sometimes recommend books that may promote healthy, plant-based diets as part of an overall approach to health and well-being. For example, Scott Jurek's autobiography, *Eat & Run*, highlights the progression of his ultrarunning career while also covering his transition to a plant-based diet (also featuring recipes).

How much does diet really affect mood and psychological well-being?

Diet has a strong relationship with mood, which is much more notable when acute nutritional needs are not met or are exceeded. For example, consuming a more consistent energy supply throughout the day leads to feeling more energetic and less fatigued, whereas infrequent or inadequate intake or consumption of refined sugars may lead to low blood sugar and subsequent symptoms including irritability, fatigue, and anxiety.

While effects on psychological well-being are not as easily identified, diet does seem to influence long-term states. For example, persons consuming a Mediterranean dietary pattern have a lower risk of depression than those consuming a Western, traditional processed diet.

Is the vegan diet equally good for everyone?

The vegan diet can be great for most people if they consume a variety of plant-based, minimally processed, and fortified foods. However, you can technically be vegan while living off of a diet consisting mostly of potato chips, Oreo cookies, pop tarts, and soda. None of these are obviously recommended for good health, and highlight the fact that a vegan diet does not automatically mean a healthy diet. Instead, vegan diets should follow general guidelines to consume a variety of foods, and ensure that any essential micronutrient needs that are not obtained through natural sources are consumed through fortified foods or supplements.

These comments all assume that the consumer is able to access and consume enough vegan products that have naturally occurring or fortified essential nutrients (mainly vitamin B12) to meet intake guidelines. Pregnant women following a vegan diet may require higher supplementation of B12 but also vegan sources of docosahexaenoic (DHA) and eicosatetraenoic (EPA) fatty acids that are less easily converted and absorbed from plant sources of omega-3 fatty acids.

What are the top dangers of veganism, and how would you recommend avoiding them?

Barriers to a healthy, balanced, and sustainable diet seem to center largely around consumer preferences, product availability, and promotion. I think people often fall into a trap they've set for themselves, where they are sparked to become a vegan or vegetarian. After this initial burst of enthusiasm and stringent diet, the variations and strains of regular life wear away at motivation and they let go of their diet altogether. I wish that people wouldn't feel that it is an all-or-nothing decision. The small choices we make every day can add up to have a huge impact.

Furthermore, the combination of a general lack of interest and skill in cooking and low access to acceptable and affordable vegan food substitutes in many areas can stifle progress towards sustainable diets. The misperception that vegan diets are expensive can also stem from this. Beans and rice are cheap plant-based staples, but a close replacement for a cheesy pizza will come at a premium.

What purchase of fifty dollars or less has improved your ability to have a healthy diet the most?

A NutriBullet! I am not sponsored in any way by the company or brand. I have just enjoyed a multitude of processing and pureeing benefits from it including smoothies, dressings, dips, and grinding flours and coffee!

Three big meals or seven small meals?

I believe this depends on the person and their food habits. If they are feeling like they "crash" throughout the day on three big meals, seven small meals might be a good solution. However, for those who prefer traditional meals and portion sizes, it may be difficult to snack on a composed meal, particularly one with meat and other sides that isn't a sandwich.

What are the two foods you'd recommend to stop eating or drastically cut out?

Eliminating, or drastically reducing, the consumption of processed and red meat would substantially benefit human health and environmental health. Consumption of red and processed meat (which has been identified as a carcinogen) increases the risk of premature mortality and morbidity from cancer, Type 2 diabetes, and cardiovascular diseases. Eliminating red and processed meat from our diets would be a win-win for humans, animals, and the environment.

What is the worst advice you hear people routinely give in the nutrition community?

I cannot stand all of the fad diets constantly circulating through the media. Many of them are not evidence based and may not be nutritionally adequate. The constant adoption and dropping of extreme diets does not support small changes towards a healthy dietary pattern that accrue into long-term behavior change and health benefits.

Not only are fad diets often ineffective in achieving long-term weight loss, but they also magnify the narrative that external beauty is what we should strive for. This usually means being thin or achieving some cookie-cutter body type. In addition to the negative effects of cycling though fad diets, the social pressures they imply can negatively impact self-perceptions, well-being, and relationships with food among dieters and non-dieters alike. Sometimes, these stressors can lead to the development of intense eating disorders while, for many, they divert attention and energy away from adopting positive behaviors that translate to long-term beneficial habits.

Low-fat vs. low-carb diet for weight loss?

This really boils down to the sources of carbohydrates, proteins, and fats in these diets. If the diet still follows the recommendations for a minimally processed, plant-based diet while remaining in the target caloric deficit for weight loss, the two are both likely to result in healthy weight loss. The appropriateness of the two diets would likely be up to individual preferences and food habits.

What is detoxification and how do you feel about the need for it?

Detoxification (detox) diets promote foods and dietary patterns that are purported to eliminate toxins that can "build up" in our bodies and negatively impact health and well-being. I do not feel that detox diets are necessary, nor is there sufficient evidence to support the use of them in short-term "cleanses."

It would be much more helpful for people if they applied a select few of these principles towards making small changes in their everyday diets. For example, reducing or eliminating highly processed foods from your diet would be a great long-term habit to adopt. Rather than "flushing" out toxins, drinking plenty of water or tea can help maintain hydration all day. Eating plenty of fruits and vegetables will, of course, provide many essential nutrients and antioxidants but will also help maintain satiety throughout the day (especially more so than in a juice form).

Intermittent fasting is often recommended in detox diets and does actually have some evidence to support short-term benefits. Some studies have found beneficial effects of fasting for metabolic and aging processes (Mattson, 2017) and potential benefits when combined with cancer treatment (Nencioni, 2018). However, based on findings from one RCT study by Trepanowski, et al. (2017), it doesn't seem that intermittent fasting is inherently better for weight loss than caloric restriction without fasting.

Breakfast or no breakfast?

Whatever works best in the context of the individual! If you aren't hungry when you wake up, and eating breakfast is a forced act that only adds unnecessary calories, leave it! If you feel hungry upon waking, or feel better if you eat breakfast, go for it. Of course, the quality of the breakfast meal and the person's needs in question could substantially change this position (e.g., pop tarts vs. steel cut oats, a person with obesity vs. diabetes).

In the past few years, what new attitude or belief has most shaped your understanding of healthy nutrition and a healthy lifestyle?

With a better understanding of the impacts our diets have on the environment, I now believe that a healthy nutrition and lifestyle support both human health but also global sustainability. The environmental impacts of our food production disproportionately impact the health and wellbeing of those in developing countries who have less power and resources. We should be mindful of how our food and lifestyle choices impact others.

What do you do when you're craving junk food?

Sometimes, I'll eat whatever I'm craving if I am not at home, whereas at home I often find another food that might satisfy my craving while still providing some nutritional value!

Sarah Pruett Soufl

Sarah is a dietitian specializing in holistic nutrition for wellness. She focuses on food and nutrition for all life stages, sports nutrition, and the disposition and development of children. Sarah has an MS in Nutritional Science and is a registered dietician.

Top quote

"Eat for physical rather than emotional reasons, rely on internal hunger and satiety cues, and give yourself unconditional permission to eat."

In the past few years, what attitude or belief has most shaped your understanding of healthy nutrition and a healthy lifestyle?

The concept of Intuitive Eating, developed by two RDs, Evelyn Tribole and Elyse Resch, has most shaped my approach to nutrition in recent years. There are ten principles that build on each other, all helping people to stop thinking of food in "good" and "bad" terms, and to start feeding themselves using the wisdom of their body, mind, and emotions. It's been helpful for people who have weight-cycled for long periods of time to come to peace with their bodies and eating.

As a quick summary, here are the principles below:

Reject the Diet Mentality—There is no such thing as "the perfect diet." Diet's generally don't work and, when you realize that, you can open up to the idea of a gentle approach to nutrition.

Honor Your Hunger—Supply your body with adequate energy and nutrients. Hunger is hunger and it won't go away because you ignore it. If you consistently allow hunger to develop, you can trigger a primal overeating drive, at which point intentions of moderate and conscious eating will be impossible to follow through. You must learn to honor these deep-rooted biological signals. Unconditional permission to eat is an important key to eating intuitively.

Make Peace with Food—Related to the diet mentality, but different. Stop fighting. Give yourself permission to eat and enjoy food. Intense feelings of deprivation build into uncontrollable cravings, binging, and guilt.

Challenge the Food Police—Anxiety related to "good" or "bad" because you ate some sugar, carbs, or ice cream has roots deep in your psyche. Eating disorders are notoriously easy to develop because worrying about food is an easy pattern to fall into for humans. Say no to guilt!

Respect Your Fullness—Learn to pay attention to the signals that you're comfortably full. Pause, observe, and learn what fullness feels like.

Discover the Satisfaction Factor—Building on the previous, the Japanese in their wisdom promote pleasure as a goal of being healthy. In our modern fast-paced lifestyle, we often overlook that pleasure and satisfaction can be found in eating slowly, gently, and with satisfaction. When you eat intuitively and without anxiety, the pleasure of eating will be a powerful force that will guide you to choose the right foods and the right quantities.

Honor Your Feelings—Find ways to resolve your psychological conflicts without relying on food. Loneliness, fear, anxiety, boredom, and anger are all feelings we experience. Food won't fix any of these feelings. It may comfort for the short term, but it won't solve the problem. If anything, eating emotionally will only make you feel worse in the long run because eating emotionally inherently means you're eating in some disbalanced way. This food disbalance will always eventually manifest in some other disbalance. Deal with the source of the emotion instead. It is much more effective.

Respect Your Body—All of our bodies are different for a variety of fundamental factors: genetics, epigenetics, microbiome, and learned habits. Be realistic about your body. That doesn't mean you can't change, but honor and cherish what you have, and let the change happen lovingly and in a way that works for your body.

Exercise—Forget harsh militant exercise and bootcamps (unless you love that). Get active and feel the difference. Shift your focus to enjoying moving your body, rather than calorie burning. Find exercise that you love, and do it at times that work for you. Do you really enjoy a 5:00 a.m. bootcamp? If you do, great. If you don't, work in exercise at times that you like and in forms that you like. Again, recall the wisdom of the Japanese and the concept of pleasure being an integral part of life.

Honor Your Health with Gentle Nutrition—It's what you eat consistently over time that matters. Take time to read about health, and gain an overall understanding of how it works. Don't fall into traps of harsh diets or promises that any one food group must be eliminated. Read, understand, reflect, and honor. The key is to think about food and nutrition enough—not too little and not too much, trusting that your body will get what it needs when you are in attunement with your internal cues and external surroundings.

Once the principles above are understood, we can further boil down intuitive eating to the three main characteristics identified by Tylka in the Intuitive Eating Assessment Scale (2006, Journal of Counseling Psychology, 53, 226-240).

Eat for physical rather than emotional reasons.

Rely on internal hunger and satiety cues.

Unconditional permission to eat.

Christina Pirello

Christina Pirello, with a Master's of Food Nutrition, is one of America's preeminent authorities on a healthier lifestyle utilizing natural and whole foods. She's made it her purpose in life to show the world that everyone can look their best and feel great, too, by learning to correctly select the best ingredients that are available. After overcoming terminal leukemia through healthy eating, and incorporating whole and unprocessed foods, she became utterly convinced of the close relationship between diet and health. Today, almost thirty years after her illness, Christina is a glowing example and inspiration about the power that food choices have and their overall impact on health and well-being. Utilizing her internationally-respected TV show, "Christina Cooks," and her many books, she is, "Changing the Health of the World One Meal at a Time."

Top quote

"You can't skip breakfast. The first food you eat, no matter the time of day, is breakfast.

What book about nutrition do you frequently recommend to friends?

There's no one book I recommend. It all depends on what someone is looking to discover. For cooking, I might recommend one of my books or, *The Self-Healing Cookbook* by Kristina Turner or *The Kind Diet* by Alicia Silverstone. If someone wants the science behind plant-based eating, I go with, *The China Study* by T. Colin Campbell.

Is the vegan diet equally good for everyone?

I think that almost everyone can benefit from a vegan diet, if it's well-balanced. From athletes to couch potatoes, and warriors to new mothers, a well-balanced vegan diet can work. That said, there are people who feel that they simply can't live well on plants alone and, for them, I would say the less animal foods, the better for their wellness (and the planet's). It's rare for a person not to be able to thrive on a balanced vegan diet.

What are the top risks of a vegan diet that you've seen, and how would you recommend avoiding those risks?

I always say that, for many people, eating a vegan diet is about what you don't do and not what you proactively do to maintain wellness. For example, many focus on not eating junk food just because it's vegan but, in fact, consuming a diet that is rich in whole, unprocessed, seasonal foods cooked appropriately for your personal health should be the focus.

I use the principles of macrobiotics and Chinese medicine to guide me. It's also essential that everyone, vegan or otherwise, exercise vigorously in order to maintain a healthy body and alleviate stress and anxiety. Studies show that regular exercise can alter moods and aid in relieving many psychological challenges.

Three big meals or seven small meals?

This one is completely personal and depends largely on your lifestyle and activity level. If someone is sedentary, I think snacking is done mostly out of boredom and not hunger. People who work in physically challenging jobs, people who are physically active, and young people still growing generally need more nutrition than people who are less so.

On the other hand, many people who "graze" all day thrive, maintain their weight, and never feel bloated or too full. In our house, we live by the age-old guideline: eat breakfast like kings, lunch like princes, and dinner like paupers. We eat a big balanced breakfast, a simpler lunch, and a light dinner. And we have a small snack before our evening workout with dinner after that.

More than deciding to snack or not, I think it's essential to stop eating 2–3 hours before you go to bed so that your body can rest and you wake up refreshed and ready to rock the day. You actually fast each and every day for 10–12 hours depending on how many hours of sleep you get and the time you eat breakfast. It's a rule we follow religiously in our house, and one of the best tips for optimizing health that there is.

What purchase of fifty dollars or less has improved your ability to have a healthy diet the most?

Several years ago, we bought a sprouting kit and have been sprouting grains and beans since then to use in various recipes.

What are the two foods you'd recommend to stop eating or drastically cut out?

If I could wave a magic wand and make a food disappear, it would be soda. This liquid poison has stolen our collective wellness in ways we can't even measure. Soda seems to create the perfect storm of sugar and chemicals that's simply lethal for our wellness.

I also think that anyone using Teflon-coated cookware should toss it out immediately. The chemical compounds have found their way into most of our waterways and most of humanity's bloodstream. Known to be carcinogenic, this non-stick coating has no place in any kitchen.

As for superfoods, I'm not a fan of the "superfood" label and deeply believe that most unrefined, whole, unprocessed, truly natural foods are all super heroes of our wellness.

What is worst advice you hear people give routinely in the nutrition community?

I think the worst advice I hear is when "experts" set down hard and fast rules for wellness. For instance, when a doctor advises that no one, no one under any circumstances, should consume any added fat in their diet; or people should eat only raw foods; or no one should take a supplement ever, etc.

That kind of extreme generalization is more about furthering someone's agenda than improving the wellness of the person in question. Each person is unique and has unique needs. Without information about an individual and their family history, and how they live, eat, and exercise, there is no place for extreme generalizations of that sort.

Low-fat vs. low-carb diet for weight loss?

I vote for neither because, in each case, the use of whole, unrefined foods and good quality fats like nuts, avocados, and extra virgin olive oil will help create wellness. When we talk about low-fat and low-carb diets, we restrict people's intake of entire groups of macro-nutrients. On top of that, you can't lump all carbohydrates and fats together. Complex carbohydrates like brown rice, quinoa, and millet are beneficial, while white flour steals our health away. Both are carbs but are not at all equal. With fats, poly and monounsaturated fats are needed by the body and aid in the absorption of fat-soluble nutrients while saturated fats, hydrogenated fats, and trans fats cause harm. So, I advocate for a balanced vegan diet with no restrictions.

Breakfast or no breakfast?

You can't skip breakfast. The first food you eat, no matter the time of day, is breakfast. In my ideal world, you would eat a complex carbohydrate breakfast (like a grain porridge) that gently brings our bodies to life and ensures stable blood sugar for the day.

In the past few years, what attitude or belief has most shaped your understanding of healthy nutrition and a healthy lifestyle?

When the World Health Organization came out with the results of a study that linked the future of our planet to a vegan diet, I was stunned. I knew that eating plants resulted in great human wellness, but I was unaware of the dramatic impact of our food choices on climate change.

What do you do when you're craving junk food?

As a former pastry chef, my cravings always tend to be sweet cravings. I always, always have small sweet treats that I make on hand in my kitchen to keep my sweet cravings in check. If I am invited out, I always volunteer to bring dessert so I can indulge. We even travel with homemade sweets. Knowing that I indulge my sweet tooth regularly makes it really easy for me to skip junk food or temptations at parties or events.

Michael Davidson

Michael Davidson, Pharm.D., A.C.N., is a doctor of pharmacy, clinical nutritionist, and phytotherapist (evidence-based herbal therapist). Even as an undergraduate studying biochemistry at UCLA, he focused on the nutritional applications, learning the core principles and underlying mechanisms of nutritional science.

While studying therapeutics, Michael developed a great interest in natural medicine, taking classes and working on projects on herbal medicine. His mission is to help people regain and maintain control of their own health and well-being so that they're able to realize their highest goals and dreams, and that their life overflows with joy and flows from them, in abundance, to those around them. Consultations with Dr. Davidson can be requested at DrMDavidson.com.

Top quote:

"There is no such thing as a diet that is equally good for everyone."

What book about nutrition do you frequently recommend to friends?

I recommend *The China Study* by T. Colin Campbell and *How Not to Die* by Michael Greger, MD and Gene Stone. Both of these books reveal the powerful impact that our lifestyle choices, especially what we choose to eat, have on our health. Both books rely on primary literature (scientific studies) to examine the relationship between diet and disease, summarizing a massive body of scientific evidence consisting of hundreds of studies to arrive at inevitable conclusions. Moreover, both of these books do a great job not only at explaining the science, but also at translating this science into easy to follow guidelines that anyone can apply to live a healthier life.

How much does diet really affect mood and psychological well-being?

There are a number of studies showing that diet has a very important effect on mood and psychological health. Some foods have been shown to have a particularly important role in promoting psychological well-being. Credible sources of nutrition information, such as nutritionfacts.org, should be referred to for examples of these and how they work. The beneficial effects of certain foods and herbs on psychological health can be explained by a variety of mechanisms such as their effect on neurotransmitters, intestinal microbiota (also known as gut flora), hormonal cascades, etc. It should be noted that all foods have an effect on the microbial environment of the human gut which, in turn, has a profound influence on psychological health and a number of organ systems.

Is the vegan diet equally good for everyone?

Prior to answering this question, I'd like to differentiate between a vegan diet and a whole food plant-based diet. It is entirely possible to have a very unhealthy diet that can still technically be called vegan. For instance, someone eating nothing but potato chips, French fries, and cookies can still claim to be eating a vegan diet. The whole food plant-based diet, on the other hand, emphasizes whole and unprocessed plant foods. So, the question should actually be is a whole food plant-based diet equally good for everyone?

The answer to that question is clearly no, due solely to the fact that there is no such thing as a diet that is equally good for everyone. Indeed, when it comes to matters of the human body, I doubt there is any substance that has an equal effect on everyone, since effects will vary depending on the individual's specific attributes such as their unique genetic makeup, physiology, health conditions, etc. Nevertheless, if the question were to be rephrased as, is the whole food plant-based diet beneficial for most people, to that I would say that there is a tremendous body of scientific literature that clearly indicates that this type of diet is beneficial for human health in general. Likewise, there's a tremendous body of scientific evidence that clearly indicates that the consumption of processed food and animal products is detrimental to human health in general.

What are the top dangers of veganism, and how would you recommend avoiding them?

There are a few pitfalls that those eating a vegan diet should avoid to protect their health. The first of these potential errors is not supplementing with vitamin B12. Although there's no reliable food source of vitamin B12, vegans are at a much higher risk of deficiency compared to omnivores, since some animal products are contaminated with bacteria that produce this vitamin. Therefore, supplementation is particularly important for vegans. For more details regarding vitamin B12 dosage and formulations, feel free to visit my website, DrMDavidson.com. for an article on this topic.

Another major health hazard is the consumption of refined oils. Vegetable oil is a particularly dangerous mixture of oils to consume in even small quantities. Processed and/or packaged foods may have large quantities of these refined oils. Although oils from other plant sources comprised of healthier fats such as olive oil, flax oil, or avocado oil are considerably less dangerous, I would recommend limiting even these oils to no more than a couple of teaspoonfuls per day (e.g., in a salad).

Finally, trying to follow a vegan diet becomes very difficult when there are more animal products and junk food in the fridge and kitchen cupboards than there are healthy foods. Replacing processed foods and animal products with whole plant foods in your kitchen should be the first step in trying to adopt a vegan lifestyle.

Three big meals or seven small meals?

The question of snacking depends on individual eating behaviors which differ from person to person. Some people find that, if they don't have a snack in between meals, they may have a tendency to overeat during the main meals. On the other hand, others may not have this problem and may find that just eating three times a day is more convenient than having to find time to snack throughout the day. Individuals with certain health conditions, such as those involving impaired sugar metabolism, may also benefit from healthy snacks in between meals. Whatever the case may be, I recommend not ignoring the need to eat or snack to the point where one feels extremely hungry, and trying not to overeat to the point where one feels excessively full.

What purchase of fifty dollars or less has improved your ability to have a healthy diet the most?

There are a number of inexpensive spices that one can add to a meal to greatly enhance its nutritional quality. For instance, just a pinch of ground cloves, or Indian gooseberries (also known as Amla) greatly enhances the nutritional content of any meal. The spices also enhance the medicinal qualities of the meal, serving as prophylactic medicine against many ailments. Amla makes it easy for me to turn even a simple meal into a nutritional powerhouse.

What are the two foods you'd recommend to stop eating or drastically cut out?

I'd recommend cutting out processed meat entirely from the diet since it's a group 1 carcinogen, which puts it in the same category as mercury and radioactive plutonium. I would also cut out fried foods since these foods often contain trans fats that can be dangerous even in small amounts.

What is worst advice you hear people give routinely in the nutrition community?

I often hear advice regarding foods that are supposedly good sources of protein. The focus on satisfying one's protein requirements is entirely misguided and flies in the face of the scientific literature, which clearly shows that vegans, vegetarians, and omnivores all get more than enough protein regardless of their diet. This is because, contrary to the popular myth, protein is actually found in all foods including fruits and vegetables. The notion that animal flesh is a better source of protein couldn't be further from the truth. While animal products have proteins that are more complete, the completeness of proteins has nothing to do with their effects on human health. In fact, the more complete proteins in animal products are far more detrimental to human health than the incomplete proteins found in whole plant foods. This point is so often confused and misunderstood that it cannot be overemphasized! On the other hand, hardly anyone talks about the importance of getting enough fiber daily, despite the fact that the vast majority of Americans are extremely deficient in this vital food component that prevents the top causes of death and disability in the U.S.

What's the top "superfood" or supplement that you recommend everyone should incorporate into their diet?

I recommend that everyone incorporate two tablespoons of ground flax seeds into their diet on a daily basis. Flax seeds are packed with nutrients, including cancer-fighting lignans and alpha-linolenic acid which serves as a precursor to the omega-3 fatty acids which are vital for cardiovascular and nervous system health. Eating them in the ground form increases the absorption of their nutrients into the body.

Low-fat vs. low-carb diet for weight loss?

I would never recommend a low-carb diet for anyone, as this type of diet is inherently dangerous to human health. The complex carbohydrates found in whole plant foods are essential to human health and well-being, so, limiting these foods can have disastrous consequences to one's health. Moreover, I would discourage people from using labels such as low-fat or low-carb since a low-fat diet can either be very healthy if it focuses on foods such as fruits and vegetables, or very unhealthy if it includes foods such as low-fat meat products or low-fat cream cheese or other processed foods. Likewise, a low–carb diet can also be very healthy if it eliminates sources of refined carbs such as sugary drinks and sweets, or very unhealthy if it eliminates whole fruit or whole grains or lentils instead. Therefore, labels such as low-fat are inherently misleading and create confusion. Eating unprocessed plant foods will very likely lead to health benefits regardless of what you call this type of diet, while eating processed foods and animal products is likely to result in negative health consequences.

What is detoxification and how do you feel about the need for it?

Detoxification is the process of eliminating toxic pollutants from the body. These pollutants accumulate in the body from a variety of primarily environmental sources, such as the air we breathe, the water we drink, what we put on our skin, and most importantly, the food we eat. Indeed, for the vast majority of people, the greatest source of exposure to environmental toxins is from the food they eat every day. Many of these harmful pollutants, such as industrial chemicals, heavy metals, pathogenic organisms, bacterial endotoxins, and many others are found at the highest concentrations in animal products such as meat, fish, dairy, and eggs. To maintain optimal functioning, the human body needs to keep levels of these toxic pollutants as low as possible. Perhaps the best way to do this is to eliminate all processed food and animal products from the diet. Another way is to not eat entirely for a time. Scientific literature indicates that fasting has a number of health benefits similar to that of a whole food plant based diet. For healthy individuals, fasting intermittently can have beneficial effects for a number of organ systems, including the immune system. Individuals with any medical conditions should consult a nutrition professional prior to fasting, especially for extended periods of time.

Breakfast or no breakfast?

There are number of scientific studies demonstrating the importance of eating breakfast. Having said that, it would be far healthier to eat nothing at all compared to eating something like bacon and eggs or the typical American breakfast. On the other hand, eating something like whole grain oatmeal with cinnamon and berries would be a very healthy way to start off the day.

In the past few years, what new attitude or belief has most shaped your understanding of healthy nutrition and and a healthy lifestyle?

What we eat everyday will have a far greater impact on our health then what we may eat on special occasions. It is not necessary to be religiously adherent to a particular diet. If we eat something unhealthy on a special occasion or due to lack of better options, there's no need to beat ourselves up about it. We should simply try to eat better the next day

What do you do when you're craving junk food?

Usually, it is when we're most hungry that we crave junk food. Once we eat something and are not as hungry, the junk food usually doesn't seem nearly as attractive anymore. Since we can only eat so much, if we fill up on healthy foods, we will not crave the unhealthy fatty or junk foods simply because we will no longer be hungry.

Instead of focusing on avoiding specific foods, I recommend focusing on eating healthy foods such as fruits, vegetables, legumes, nuts, seeds, mushrooms, and whole grains. If we eat enough of these healthy foods, they will effectively replace the detrimental foods that we may otherwise crave since we will no longer have room for much else. Moreover, we can satisfy the craving for a specific junk food by eating a healthy food with similar characteristics as the food we're craving. For instance, if the craving is for a dessert or sweet, we can instead eat a sweet fruit such as a date or a banana. If the craving is for something fatty and creamy like butter, we can instead eat something like an avocado or a nut butter. If the craving is for a crunchy and cheesy junk food like cheesy chips, we can instead eat raw cauliflower sprinkled with nutritional yeast.

If no healthy foods are available, we can distract ourselves from the craving by focusing on a different activity. The most effective type of diversion will depend on the individual, but may include things like reading, taking a jog, listening to an audiobook, breathing exercises, listening to music, speaking on the phone, working on a project, etc. I'd recommend doing something that you find enjoyable or fascinating since, the more engrossing this activity is, the more effective this technique will be at distracting you from the craving. Removing triggers such as junk food in your own home should be done, as well, since it's much more difficult to eat what you don't have readily available.

Andrea Smoko

Prior to her current career as a Registered Dietitian and Lactation Consultant, Andrea worked as chef and co-owner of a small restaurant in Northern Wisconsin with her husband of twenty-eight years. She attended the Culinary Institute of America in New York to fulfill her dream of being a chef. She returned to school thirteen years later to finish with a certificate in Dietetics and become registered as a dietitian/nutritionist.

Top quote

"As a child growing up, we were taught that 'you are what you eat.' This has always made a lot of sense to me and holds more truth the older I get. It is my go-to phrase."

What book about nutrition do you frequently recommend to friends?

101 Foods That Could Save Your Life, by David Grotto, RD, LDN. It is written by a fellow dietitian and contains a wealth of interesting information on literally 101 food items like nuts, seeds, grains, fruits, and vegetables. The information is presented in easy to browse paragraphs with topic headings that offer biological properties of the food, growing conditions, where it originated and how it found its way into the western diet, historical anecdotes and uses, health benefits specific to medical conditions, and tips on selection, storage, preparation, and serving. Each food entry is accompanied by a recipe using that food as well.

Is the vegan diet equally good for everyone?

I could not recommend that everyone follow a vegan diet, nor do I believe it is possible. As infants, we rely on milk from our mothers to sustain life and for healthy growth. So, our first food of life, itself, defies the practice of veganism. Beyond that, there are a couple of key nutrients needed for optimal childhood growth and adult health maintenance where animal products seem to provide a more reliable source, especially iron and vitamin B12. Sure, there are supplements available to fill in where nutritional gaps exist, but they can be costly for some, or difficult to take and remember to take. Furthermore, our bodies absorb nutrients best through real food sources over laboratory forms.

With this being said, however, I believe that we would all benefit from adopting some of the concepts of eating <u>less</u> meat and animal products and <u>more</u> plant-based foods as we enter adulthood and live out the remainder of our lives. The impact that would have on reducing the rate of heart disease, cancer, hypertension, and other chronic diseases would be incredibly positive, not to mention the environmental impact of fewer feedlots and poultry farms reducing pollution.

Three big meals or seven small meals?

It makes more sense to eat several small meals and snacks than three large ones. There are several reasons why. Blood glucose levels remain steadier, thereby increasing the body's physical and mental performance and reducing inflammatory response. Digestion is better facilitated when it is not insulted with large amounts of food to process and so is the ability to be mindful of what and how much one eats, which is what we should all strive for.

The confusion about whether or not snacking is healthy is in how the word is used. Many consider a snack not as a small amount of food eaten, but rather as the type of food eaten, thanks to the food manufacturing industry and the way they market their products as 'snack foods.' I promote snacking between meals when you actually feel a little pang of hunger (not boredom) and it is a couple of hours until your usual meal time. A snack is a small amount of food and it is wise to include at least two food groups (i.e., cheese and whole grain crackers, yogurt and fruit, or veggie strips and hummus, for example).

What are the two foods you'd recommend to stop eating or drastically cut out?

Cheap sliced white bread and puffed cheese snacks. Both are highly processed to the point of not even qualifying as actual food, both are addictive and seemingly very popular. It is a shame that manufacturers of infant foods have produced a product similar to puffed cheese that they refer to as 'Baby Cheetos,' and that young parents believe it is a good product to offer their children. Instead, it is just getting poor eating habits off to an early start.

Conversely, since the typical western diet is essentially void of natural food sources rich in vitamin D, and not everyone lives roughly within 1,000 miles of the equator, I advocate for vitamin D supplementation for a large population (of all ages) that doesn't see much sunshine.

What is worst advice you hear people give routinely in the nutrition community?

The worst advice is to offer no advice at all about the need to accompany any dietary regimen with a commitment to a whole lifestyle change that includes physical activity. To consider such a one-dimensional strategy as to simply follow today's popular diet, or to take a supplement with exaggerated claims to melt body fat, for example, is misleading and will likely result in failure. It is important for any eating plan to be sustainable, or else one is faced with ending up worse off than they started if their goals are unrealistic, or their lifestyle hasn't changed.

Low-fat vs. low-carb diet for weight loss?

Weight loss is a matter of ingesting fewer calories than one expends for body mechanics and activities of daily living. Low carbohydrate diets, while they may show promising weight loss results, can overwork the body's renal system, are inadequate in some key nutrients, and are difficult to sustain. Low fat diets are often higher in sugars to increase their palatability and often fail because the body's satiety triggers are bypassed by additives that go unrecognized with normal digestion.

Breakfast or no breakfast?

Yes! Our digestive system needs to be stimulated after being without for a lengthy period of time or else it will enter into 'starvation mode' to conserve energy. In the morning is when our body's metabolism is ready to work most efficiently, but it needs a signal from ingested food to trigger it.

In the past few years, what attitude or belief has most shaped your understanding of healthy nutrition and a healthy lifestyle?

As a child growing up, I was taught 'you are what you eat.' This has always made a lot of sense to me and holds more truth the older I get. It is my go-to phrase.

What do you do when you're craving junk food?

I usually respond to these cravings without too much guilt because I realize they are infrequent and temporary. In general, an eating plan that is normally balanced with a healthy foods routine, established as habit for many years, is rarely in danger of an occasional slip-up. If I become concerned that these occasions happen too frequently, I know I need to revisit my goals for living a healthy life.

Mauvis Miller

Mauvis has a clinic in North County San Diego called iNourish, a body-mind center. She educates clients on how they should not separate or differentiate between the mind and the body, and how this connection is used as a tool to find "the root cause" of issues via a systemology and history questionnaire. Mauvis has an education in traditional and holistic nutrition from institutions such as Cornell University, the Institute for Psychology of Eating, and MiraCosta College.

Top quote

"Water, water, water is a great cleanse."

What book about nutrition do you frequently recommend to friends?

I have a few depending on the client's needs but one book, well, two books are on my desk that I frequently reference and share with my clients. One is *Staying Healthy with Nutrition* by Elson M. Haas, MD and Buck Levin, Ph.D., RD. The other book is *The Worlds Healthiest Foods* by George Mateljan. In George's book, he breaks down each food by the best foods to eat according to nutrient density and the way to cook them while keeping as many nutrients intact for better absorption. Each book shows how to use nutrition as medicine with regard to certain ailments and the two together are my bible and dictionary.

How much does diet really affect mood and psychological well-being?

It's everything. Food can make or break you. We eat to nourish our bodies which ultimately affects our minds because there is no separation of the two. More and more of today's science and clinical studies are bringing forth proof on how the mind and the body are interrelated and how we need to focus on both when we seek to prevent and even reverse ailments. The old saying was, "You are what you eat" and that has been updated to a more violent truth, "You are what you digest."

Is the vegan diet equally good for everyone? Why or why not?

Veganism is a movement and there are so many times when I talk with someone and they claim they are vegan. Eight out of ten don't know the true reason of veganism. I share and explain some history on what it means to be a true vegan and then throw in the difference of being "plant based." There are quite a bit of AhHa moments that ring true with their choice and actually the majority of them then change their preference to being just "plant based." I also do simple tests and other questionnaires to see what kind of diet they are suited for the best.

What are the top dangers of veganism, and how would you recommend avoiding them?

Who's to say? You can get all the nutrients the body needs by adding supplements to a vegan diet if one is determined to become or even stay a vegan.

Three big meals or seven small meals?

That depends on the client's goals. Is it to lose weight, to gain weight, or to just be healthy? I also stress on listening to the body and whether there is any exercise part of the lifestyle? There are so many ways to answer this question hence the need for personalized and individualized protocols.

What purchase of fifty dollars or less has improved your ability to have a healthy diet the most?

A five dollar journal, a free walk in the park, a twenty dollar cooking lesson on nutrient dense cooking, and a plethora of DIY YouTube videos on meditation.

What are the two foods you'd recommend to stop eating or drastically cut out?

Sugar, because it fires off the same part of the brain as when someone is on heroin and it feeds cancer, among other dire straits. Red meat, because the AHA (American Heart Association) now claims on their website that eating red meat may cause heart disease. However, they have recipes on the same website that contain red meat.

What is worst advice you hear people give routinely in the nutrition community?

Someone is always giving advice, yet it may not necessarily be specific or tailored to whom they are giving it to. This "one size fits all approach" is often a sign of "bad advice."

What's the top "superfood" or supplement that you recommend everyone should incorporate into their diet?

Apples because they are nutrient dense, and they have their own case. You can tote them anywhere. They give you energy when you're at a 2:00 p.m. slump and they have plenty of fiber.

What is detoxification and how do you feel about the need for it?

Water, water, water is a great cleanser. If you're not drinking plenty of water, then you're retoxing.

Breakfast or no breakfast?

Breakfast helps set you up for the day, just like exercise and meditation. Yes, to all three. Oh, and plates should be 80 percent raw and 20 percent cooked. One slice of wheat toast, fresh avocado, fresh tomato, and maybe a little raw crushed garlic if you're brave. Topped with balsamic and EVOO. (Just an example!)

In the past few years, what new attitude or belief has most shaped your understanding of healthy nutrition and a healthy lifestyle?

Deep breaths, and having a grateful and happy attitude every day, and also as you sit and feast over healthy meals with others while savoring each bite.

What do you do when you're craving junk food?

Its kinda rare since I grew up sucking on lemons. In elementary when lunch was served I would flip over my little square cake dessert because I did not like frosting and just eat from the bottom up. Friends would make fun of me but I just could not fathom how they could eat all that sugar and like it. I don't have a sweet or salty tooth. And eating anything with sugar will five me a tummy ache and possible headache. If I do crave something, it will be like a dark chocolate peanut butter cup. Costco has these tiny ones that are half the size of a regular Reece's plus its 80 percent less sugar, so, all I taste is the bitter cocoa and creamy peanut butter. Frozen, please!

Dina Colman

Dina Colman is an author, health coach, and the founder of Four Quadrant Living. After Dina's sister was diagnosed with Stage 3 breast cancer, and being told that she had an 87 percent chance of getting the disease herself, Dina left her high-tech corporate career and went back to school. She earned a master's degree in holistic health education, learning how to reduce her odds of getting cancer by changing how she lived her life. Twenty years later, Dina and her sister are both cancer free.

Dina now shares what she learned in order to inspire others around the world to live happier and healthier lives. She has her own private practice, works as a wellness coach at Kaiser Permanente, and is author of award-winning *Four Quadrant Living: Making Healthy Living Your New Way of Life* (Oct 2013).

Top quote

"I believe that a part of health is pleasure. Always stressing about what we eat is not healthy."

What book about nutrition do you frequently recommend to friends?

Michael Pollan's *Food Rules*. Simple and to the point.

What purchase of fifty dollars or less has improved your ability to have a healthy diet the most?

My electric teapot for my daily green tea.

What is good advice for someone who is trying to lose weight?

The two best pieces of advice for losing weight from a behavior change standpoint is 1) to understand your "why;" and 2) to take baby steps (so that it becomes a way of life rather than a quick fix). Research shows that the more people can articulate why they want to make a change, the more likely they are to make the change. It is not about losing the weight, it is about the value you attach to being at your desired weight. For some, it could be to fit into the clothes in their closet, for others it can be about health concerns like diabetes, and for others it can be to be a role model for their children or grandchildren.

Remembering your why can help you make the changes to reach your goal. Taking baby steps is important because too often people will go from 0 to 60, such as not working out at all to going to the gym five days a week, or having three sodas a day to none. This may be doable in the short term, but is not a long-term solution which is why people go up and down with their weight. The idea is to start with steps that feel doable and build on it from there so that it is a way of life rather than something they are doing temporarily.

When patients come to see you for nutritional advice, what are some things they hear that usually surprise them?

I believe that a part of health is pleasure. There is the term, orthorexia, the unhealthy obsession with healthy eating. When I first learned about nutrition, I was probably bordering orthorexia, watching everything I put in my mouth. However, there can come a point where this isn't healthy. Always stressing about what we eat is not healthy. The key is that when you have a treat, enjoy it fully. Have that piece of cake, but really taste it, see it, feel it. Eating mindfully rather than on autopilot will help you feel more satiated with less.

In the past few years, what attitude or belief has most shaped your understanding of healthy nutrition and a healthy lifestyle?

My book, *Four Quadrant Living: Making Healthy Living Your New Way of Life*, is based on the idea that there is more to our health than just the body quadrant. In this country, we focus on the body quadrant (diet and exercise) when we talk about health, but that is only one-quarter of the story. There are three other quadrants that impact our health: mind, relationships, and environment. We may be eating well and exercising, but we cannot truly be healthy if our mind is stressed, our relationships are toxic, and our world is sick. Every day we make choices that impact our health—not just the foods we eat, but also the products we use, the exercise we get, the stress we allow, the people we surround ourselves with, and the environment we live in.

Stephanie Papadakis

Stephanie Papadakis, N.C. is a Certified Holistic Nutrition Consultant, AIP Certified Coach, and Certified Grief Recovery Specialist living in the San Francisco Bay Area. Having experienced way too much loss before the age of thirty—the three most important women in her life getting diagnosed with autoimmune diseases, suffering years of digestive issues of her own, and realizing queer nutritionists are few and far between—she went back to school in her mid-thirties to obtain a certificate from Bauman College.

Stephanie now runs Gut of Integrity, an inclusive holistic nutrition and wellness consulting business that specializes in everything from one-on-one consults, corporate wellness workshops, grief recovery classes, and restaurant menu consultations. She currently works with clients, in-person and virtually, to help address health imbalances caused by autoimmune diseases, hormonal issues, poor digestive health, SIBO, stress, and grief. Find her at gutofintegrity.com.

Top quote

"Conventional foods really are less nutritious than organic foods."

What book about nutrition do you frequently recommend to friends?

The 21-Day Sugar Detox by Diane Sanfilippo. This book changed my life by helping me to cut out sugar. The book gives you choices to meet you where you're at in the process, and by the end of 21 days you feel really good, so good you want to continue keeping refined sugar at bay. Plus, the recipes are delicious and most are fairly simple to make.

What purchase of fifty dollars or less has improved your ability to have a healthy diet the most?

A food scale. I'm not one to measure out my food, but I do measure out my animal protein. We tend to overeat protein in this country. You'll see anything from 8–32 ounce. steaks, half chickens, or racks of lamb on restaurant menus. A good measure for the amount of protein per meal, if you don't have a scale, is the size of your palm and the height of a deck of cards. If you do have a scale, 3–6 ounces is good for most people, depending on height and weight, of course.

Once I began weighing my protein, I noticed that I was less painfully full after meals. I also replaced the protein I wasn't eating with more vegetables. If you're bloated and full for a long time after meals, try getting a food scale and seeing if that makes a difference.

What are some typical challenges that your vegan clients experience, and how would you recommend addressing them?

I think the hardest challenge for vegan clients is using food as true medicine because there are so many nutrient-dense foods that are not included in a vegan diet. I work with a lot of clients with autoimmune diseases, and the vegan and vegetarian clients are usually the last to see changing results. I had one vegan client who wanted her symptoms to go away so badly she adopted a modified AIP diet by adding cold-water fish and marine collagen. She saw vast improvements in her symptoms in just a couple of weeks, but she ultimately had a hard time reconciling her guilt from eating fish and went back to eating vegan. Her symptoms came back but she was happy to be living her truth again. Personally, I support my clients' needs and beliefs and do my best to create a personalized nutrition plan that is aligned with their beliefs.

What is the worst advice you hear people give routinely in the nutrition community?

When I hear the nutrition community say that juice cleanses are healthy for you, I cringe. Fresh-pressed juice can be great for someone who has a hard time chewing food or has a low appetite due to chemotherapy and/or radiation and needs an easy way to get nutrients into their body (and I would recommend to dilute the juice so the sugar doesn't spike insulin levels and crashes). But drinking straight juice for one or more days can do the following to your body: 1) go into starvation mode so even if you lose a few pounds, you'll gain them right back once you start eating food again; 2) spike your blood sugar so you'll constantly be crashing and burning throughout the day; 3) not provide enough nutrients because the nutrients in juice deplete the longer the juice sits on the shelf; and 4) put your body into fight or flight response (i.e., stress mode) because it doesn't know where the next meal is coming from. I say no to juice cleanses every time.

What is good advice for someone who is trying to lose weight?

Instead of thinking about losing weight, think about making a lifestyle change and forming new habits. Habits take 21 days to form, so, if you can get through that time, you're in the clear. Losing weight is not just about exercise, it's also about changing what foods you eat, your stress levels, the amount of sleep you get each night, alcohol consumption, and rest and relaxation. If you focus on all of these components, and work on making a habit out of each of them, the changes will come and the weight will fall off.

When patients come to see you for nutritional advice, what are some things they hear that usually surprise them?

Conventional foods really are less nutritious than organic foods! This depletion of nutrients is due to the "dilution effect" which includes plant breeding, irrigation, and intensive utilization of synthetic fertilizers which causes nutrient depletion of the soil through runoff (this also extends to the animals that use the conventional crops for feed). In addition, synthetic fertilizers, due to their high nitrogen content, can create high levels of plant nitrates, which can harm the GI tract.

When you hear that many people have egg allergies or sensitivities, it's usually to the egg white and not the yolk. Lysozyme enzyme in egg whites is very good at breaking down bad bacteria and it does a great job of transporting the bad bacteria across the gut barrier and into the bloodstream, which can stimulate the immune system, stirring up allergies and sensitivities. This is especially true for those with autoimmune diseases, which is why it's recommended to avoid eggs until the autoimmune disease is in remission.

In the past few years, what attitude or belief has most shaped your understanding of healthy nutrition and a healthy lifestyle?

Stress management! The biggest thing I've learned over the last few years is that stress plays a bigger role in nutrition and lifestyle than food and exercise. I've had so many clients come in with autoimmune diseases that were triggered by a big life-changing event—like the death of a loved one, divorce, job loss, or big move, or more job responsibilities that led to loss of personal time and prioritizing work over self care. Such heavy stress places a severe physical burden on the adrenals, the liver, and the endocrine system but, even more so, it really takes a toll on the gut-brain axis, impairing mood and digestion. It's really important to support the whole body with the proper nutrients, lots of sleep, moderate movement, and stress management and relaxation techniques. It takes looking at the whole picture to help the whole body reset and function properly.

Sasha Williams

Sasha Williams is a retired semi-professional dancer, vegan activist, and nutritionist. She ended fifteen years in dancing after being diagnosed with cancer, and pursued her education in holistic health and wellness. She also became a professional natural bodybuilding and fitness expert, focusing on the vegan diet. Sasha operates her private fitness consulting firm, Food Medicine Life. She published her first vegan cookbook in 2017.

Top quote

"Lying about the calories you eat doesn't put you in a good place to start a health improvement journey."

What book about nutrition do you frequently recommend to friends?

Oh, there are a great number of books to recommend, for sure, but what I notice is that for attention span where nutrition is involved you need to find a book that is an easy but scientifically informative book that puts across points with a foundation built on studies and facts. So, it's a tie between *How Not to Die* and *The China Study,* for sure. Most folks err on the side of *How Not to Die* for whatever reason.

What purchase of fifty dollars or less has improved your ability to lead a healthy diet the most?

Probably of late (based on the budget), I would say my air fryer. It's really almost eliminated the need for using oil at all in my life. I live on the road permanently and only have a stove and a grill with me. My rig has no oven. So this is a great substitute. I'm able to make my own seitan while on the road which is pretty epic when you're in the deep south and there is hardly anywhere to find a block of tofu! If there was a larger budget, I'd say my Japanese hand-forged knives but they're $350–$500 per knife. They make cooking beautiful, fun, meditative, and efficient.

What are some typical challenges that your vegan clients experience, and how would you recommend addressing them?

Longer-term vegans are really the best at being WF based, so they have less issues. My "new" vegans of the last five years or so have become vegan during a food revolution and they are extremely addicted to processed or junk vegan food as it is so readily available. Training mindsets to think back to whole foods is extremely difficult as people nowadays feel personally offended by someone questioning their nutritional choices.

Most folks want to hear they can live off of vegan mac and cheese and still see results and be healthy, which is sad and leads to a lot of hard talks about truth with my clients. Honestly, it's all about food addiction, breaking the unhealthy cycles, and stepping out and saying, "I'm not going to be another number for the medical industry." Saving animals and the planet is one thing but, when your products contain palm oil that is killing orangutans and decimating their habitats, how vegan are you? I stand my ground with my clients. They hire me to hear the truth and I've never been a shrinking violet . If you're paying me for my opinion, you'll get it!

What is the worst advice you hear people give routinely in the nutrition community?

Well, there are a lot of WFPB vegan nutrition advisors or community members who will hate on soy. Now, while there are a lot of reasons to ensure you're getting a reasonable amount of QUALITY soy in your diet without going overboard, there are a lot of folks lacking in the science who make claims. One of them is that soy will give you cancer. Also, the fact that protein doesn't matter and that it is in everything. While almost true, protein is required as an important macronutrient and to reach satiety. Living on fruit or a diet full of simple carbohydrates has negative impacts for us all. Those are my two pet peeves. And really, everyone is a know-it-all these days without any backup. If you take the time to read the science behind the foods we eat, it becomes evident that "everything in moderation" is the key as opposed to utilizing fad diets.

What is good advice for someone who is trying to lose weight?

Definitely acknowledging that you need to incorporate exercise in your daily life as well as reducing stress and inflammation. Most people run out of steam midweek and fall off the wagon. This is usually due to an unmanageable schedule or lack of consistency. It's all mind over matter with getting a good habit formed and you're nothing without rest and hydration. The most irritable clients or the ones that fall off the wagon the most are simply the ones who really do not want to do the work. They are lazy, lack discipline, or didn't have any previous healthy regimes in their life. Start with the basics to improve your mood, motivation, and self respect and then go for the tough "dieting" and fitness plans.

When patients come to see you for nutritional advice, what are some things they hear that usually surprise them?

Usually I end up pointing out a few things: They don't eat enough of the good stuff and they're actually in a relative starvation mode. Most of my clients complain after working with me that they can't eat as much as I'd like them too. Ahhhh, the protein/fiber lesson!

Lying about the calories you eat doesn't put you in a good place to start a health improvement journey. Being honest about how much and what types of food you put on your plate and in your mouth is paramount. Portion distortion is a real issue for a lot of people who are borderline binge eating because of emotional issues. Food is mood for a lot of people and the types of clients I have that hear this speech are usually food addicts using calories to cope with emotional issues.

Not all "chemicals" in foods are bad or dangerous. There is a real hate on for chemicals in food which, for a lot of high-quality items, are just the scientific name for things like lemon juice. Nothing frustrates me more than people who jump onto the organic and non-gmo whole foods bandwagon from a place of utter lack of knowledge. If you are worried about ingesting non-natural foods, you also need to put down soda, alcohol, ground meat, tobacco, refined products, etc. I preach the dirty dozen and avoidance of processed foods when possible but the folks who are all upset about "chemicals" are usually, themselves, filled with them from prescription medications, topical beauty products, etc. I'm sure you can tell this is a sore spot with me.

In the past few years, what attitude or belief has most shaped your understanding of healthy nutrition and a healthy lifestyle?

I've definitely come back to my roots with meditation and mental health first. As a professional natural bodybuilder, whose worth is often related to how many abs you have during the year, you can sustain a lot of emotional damage from having to keep up an image that isn't true to who you are or who you want to be inside. Being over the top with nutritional ideals, fitness regimes, etc., can leave a person feeling hollow and like they'll never be good enough. I practice a good heap of self-acceptance in my work and start most of my clients off with a long assessment of their self esteem, their 30,000 foot view of themselves, and WHY they want to (or think they need to) make changes to their routine. Healthy living begins and ends in consciousness. If our minds are not right, we will never be in a place to truly honor our bodies.

Mark Simon

Mark studied nutrition for a very long time. Thirty-seven years ago, he decided to go on a vegan diet. Then his wife ended up with breast cancer and, unfortunately, he didn't know enough at the time to help her. Since then, he has learned many things.

Top Quote

"Don't eat processed foods and don't eat junk foods."

What book about nutrition do you frequently recommend to friends?

One of the best books available right now is *How Not to Die* by Michael Gregor. His website, nutritionfacts.org, is probably the best source of information. I've read about 100 books on the subject and his book lays out the subject extensively.

Another book, which was really important for me as a vegan for many years, is *Dr. Neal Barnard's Program for Reversing Diabetes: The Scientifically Proven System for Reversing Diabetes without Drugs*. I had issues with blood sugar stability and was developing Type 2 diabetes.

If one really wants to go deep into the spirituality aspects, I recommend the books by Dr. Gabriel Cousens.

What purchase of fifty dollars or less has improved your ability to have a healthy diet the most?

A recent purchase I made was a ceramic-coated wok called "Green Pan" and I use it all the time for cooking! It was around thirty dollars. It makes cooking really quick and easy. Nothing sticks to it!

Also, supplementation with algae oil made a big difference – it's a great source of DHA. Converting ALA into EPA and DHA can be an issue for a lot of vegans.

What are some typical challenges that your vegan clients experience, and how would you recommend addressing them?

First of all, a common challenge is being hungry, not getting enough calories, and losing weight. Because many vegans end up with low fat intake, the overall energy intake is pretty low. I recommend adding potatoes for extra calories and rice. I also warn people not to fill up too much on vegetables. There's just not enough calories there. If you're physically and mentally active, you have to eat enough food to meet your caloric intake requirement. When you readjust from really high fat-type foods to foods that are not energy dense in comparison, caloric deficiency can result. If you switch a diet quickly, you need to create a whole new rhythm in the digestive tract, so pay attention to these changes.

Another challenge is that when people start eating more fiber and fruits and vegetables, there can some digestive issues. To battle this, you have to follow some principles of food combining. People's sensitivity to various food combinations varies, but you can keep this as a tool in your toolkit if you have digestive issues. You can google "food combining" to easily find more information on this subject. Some people may have stronger digestion than others and can handle more complex kinds of meals but, overtime, this can change, so, it's important to keep food combining in mind. Food is only as good as we can digest it and eliminate it. One of the biggest problems with meat and animal flesh in the diet is that a lot of it becomes undigested in the colon, which can feed various bacteria, leading to undesirable consequences.

There are a lot of challenges coming from internal fear, as well, like are you getting enough protein, iron, etc., coupled with the projected fear from friends and family. On top of that, social interactions can be a little challenging, when you're eating differently from the rest of the people around you. Eating should be an enjoyable, relaxing activity, so this fear around food can be unhealthy and lead to nervousness.

What is the worst advice you hear people give routinely in the nutrition community?

Probably one of the worst pieces of advice that I hear is to go on a ketogenic diet. It's not healthy at all (perhaps with the exception of a few special cases where an interventional diet is necessary).

The other bad advice I hear a lot is to eat more protein. For instance, when it comes to aging, a particular amino acid called "methionine" is now the number one hypothesis for causing aging. It's found the most in chicken and fish. Packing in excessive amounts of protein exposes you to large quantities of this amino acid. Instead, consider a balanced diet with an appropriate amount of protein, not "as much as possible." An appropriate amount of protein intake is .3g/kg, which also corresponds to the RDI for people with kidney issues.

As far as building muscle, you're still better off with protein amounts that are on the lower side of the spectrum. Muscles take a long time to build, and muscles aren't pure protein anyway. They're made from tissue that is composed of a lot of different elements. When you're doing weight lifting and physical exercises, you should focus on getting enough calories in a balanced way and don't overemphasize protein. Another point to keep in mind is that there's a difference between a healthy diet and a diet that will lead to the most rapid muscle gain. Certain diets that highly emphasize protein after weight lifting may lead to faster results, but this may not necessarily be healthy in the long run.

In general, we need to get away from the simple views such as, "meat is for protein and protein is for muscle" and "milk is calcium and calcium is for bones." Instead, the focus should be on balance overall.

What is good advice for someone who is trying to lose weight?

The basic concept of keeping fat at a minimum is important.

For weight loss, also definitely follow food combining principles. (For efficient digestions, and avoidance of gastro-intestinal issues which could trigger unbalanced eating and eating at the wrong times.) There's a normal rhythm with the digestive tract. If you have digestive disturbances, it could cause one to go to the bathroom too often, or feel pangs of hunger, etc.

Food combining enters into this because it affects how one's gut feels, and it affects how food passes through the gut. You want nutrients to be released evenly overtime. Our gut is intimately interconnected with our brain. The number of nerves in the GI tract is huge. This is why some people say, "the gut is the real brain" and the brain is "an accessory." These systems evolve intimately and closely surround the functioning of the gut.

Additionally, don't eat processed foods, don't eat junk foods, and the weight will come off on its own.

Colleen Carney Ruge

Colleen has worked in the healthcare industry for over fifteen years teaching communities across the country a logical and practical approach to nutrition. She has worked with thousands of people over the years and has seen major transformations in health and lifestyle.

Colleen has also worked in a chiropractic office as the staff nutritionist and business manager for six years. She understands the challenges practitioners face with implementing nutrition solutions and wants to help more practitioners be successful with a simple, effective way to get results for their patients. Colleen is a Certified Clinical Nutritionist.

Top Quote

"Many vegan diets use soy products to replace animal products, such as Tofurky! Such soy products are a cheap replacement for protein and they are inflammatory. Too much soy can be harmful to your health."

Is the vegan diet equally good for everyone?

Vegan diets can be very healthy and easier on digestion if done correctly, however, many vegans eat too many carbohydrates and not enough leafy green vegetables, healthy fats, and protein. It is more difficult to get a good blend of amino acids on an all-Vegan/Vegetarian diet, so, plant based protein shakes are an important recommendation. People also need to be very thoughtful in their food planning and preparation to make sure they are covering all the bases of nutrition.

What is the biggest "wrong advice" that you hear regularly when it comes to vegan nutrition and a vegan lifestyle?

A lot of vegan/vegetarians are told to eat beans and legumes for their source of protein but those foods also have a high fiber and carb content and can create weight gain or carb overload which may not be desired, especially if you are diabetic. You still need a well-balanced diet with a variety of nutrients.

What's the single piece of nutritional advice (vegan-related or not) that you find yourself giving over and over to people?

Being fit and/or thin doesn't mean a person is healthy. Taking care of your body and vital organs should be the focus of any diet and healthy lifestyle. 80 percent (if not more) of your body composition is determined by what you eat. Eating nutrient-dense foods will help your body perform better and maintain the right weight for each individual.

What book about nutrition do you frequently recommend to friends?

I don't usually recommend books because they are very lengthy and sometimes confusing to the average reader. Also, there is too much focus on the problems and not the solution; however, the concepts from many anti-inflammatory food diets and books apply to everyone and provide good roadmaps to better health. *The Pure 28-Day Cleanse and Nutrition Guide* I helped write for Nutragen is a great starting point for general health and nutrition. This program includes the key concepts from many diet and nutrition sources.

What purchase of fifty dollars or less has improved your ability to have a healthy diet the most?

Water! Water! Water! Many health conditions and inflammatory responses are directly related to dehydration and most people are dehydrated. Water is vital to good health and weight loss. This was my first answer because water is actually free and it makes a big difference. I also think everyone needs a single-cup blender. Some are expensive but I buy the Bella Cucina one which is around thirty dollars.

What are some typical challenges that your vegan clients experience, and how would you recommend addressing them?

Many of the vegan/vegetarian clients I have worked with do not get enough variety of nutrients in their diets. They run out of ideas for what to eat and tend to eat the same things over and over or they just eat a ton of carbs. Experimenting with new foods and recipes is very important. Being thoughtful in meal planning, and spicing things up, makes a diet and lifestyle changes more fun too!

What is the worst advice you hear people give routinely in the nutrition community?

Many vegan diets use soy products to replace animal products, such as Tofurky! Such soy products are a cheap replacement for protein and they are inflammatory. Too much soy can be harmful to your health. You do not need to replace things like dairy, chicken nuggets, etc., you just need to stop eating these processed foods altogether (albeit gradually for some, due to behavioral reasons).

What is good advice for someone who is trying to lose weight?

You really are what you eat! Your body knows what to do with real food nutrients. If you eat a diet full of processed foods, preservatives, and chemicals, not only will you be sick, it will be much harder to maintain a healthy weight. Food toxins are stored in fat, so, eating foods that the body knows how to break down, utilize, and eliminate properly is essential to weight loss. I still hear people saying that you can eat whatever you want if you are burning it off with exercise. The calorie in, calorie out concept does not work, especially as you get older.

When patients come to see you for nutritional advice, what are some things they hear that usually surprise them?

Here are a few. Coffee is okay if you drink it black and only have a cup or two a day. Don't calorie count, just make what you eat count. Don't eat if you are not hungry but always have a healthy balanced meal to start the day (does not have to be at

8:00 a.m.). Whether you like them or not, leafy green vegetables are the cure to most diseases, so, you must eat them! Greens provide natural vitamins, minerals, anti-oxidants, etc., that is why they are so strongly linked to disease prevention.

In the past few years, what attitude or belief has most shaped your understanding of healthy nutrition and a healthy lifestyle?

After fifteen years of educating both practitioners and patients, I have realized that it is very important to make lifestyle changes realistic. It is not what we know as healthcare practitioners, it is more about what we now know people will and will not do. There is no one size fits all diet and we have to be conscious and considerate when helping people with change. I am not an extremist when it comes to being healthy, and I show people how to live healthy lives but also have fun and indulge every once in a while. There are remedies for all bad choices.

P.S. When you fall off your diet, get right back on. There is no such thing as cheating. If you make bad choices, then you must make good ones.

Tristan Thibodeau

After earning her Bachelor's Degree in Dietetics, Master's Degree in Human Nutrition, and the certification as an Integrative Nutrition Health Coach from the Institute for Integrative Nutrition, Tristan founded Honest to Goodness Health to create a vehicle of healthcare that aligned with her values, which includes an appreciation and understanding of bio-individuality, and a holistic approach to health that includes an evaluation of lifestyle, relationships, emotional state, and career, and how these can affect an individual's health.

Top quote

"Transitioning into a vegan diet does take diligent planning and attention to ensure a diverse and balanced diet."

What book about nutrition do you frequently recommend to friends?

This might come as a shock, but I never offer unsolicited advice or input about the diet of another individual unless I am explicitly asked. Nutrition is such a personal facet to one's lifestyle, so, I think it's important to individualize as much as is possible based on the traits of the individual and their current lifestyle. However, I do have favorite books on a few topics that I myself have found extremely helpful.

For any individual, but especially women, who may be struggling in their relationship with food, I highly recommend *Eating in the Light of the Moon* by Dr. Anita Johnson. This book is a phenomenal resource that uses storytelling and folklore to describe some of the more difficult aspects of disordered eating in a way that is juxtaposed to any other approach on the topic I have found. Dr. Johnson is a pioneer in eating psychology and offers readers a refreshing take on how to honor your body and its needs through food and emotional intelligence.

For those who want to learn to eat in a way that will prevent most of the lifestyle-based diseases that are prevalent today such as hypercholesterolemia, diabetes, and heart disease, I highly recommend *The Blood Sugar Solution* by Dr. Mark Hyman, Director for Functional Medicine at the Cleveland Clinic. This book is a phenomenal step-by-step approach to helping you revamp your lifestyle and address your own unique health issues or short-comings through a scientific, yet accessible method.

What purchase of fifty dollars or less has improved your ability to have a healthy diet the most?

What a fun question to consider! I would have to say either a digital food scale or a liter sized stainless-steel water bottle.

I use my food scale to help me be realistic with my serving sizes. I think it's an extremely valuable experience for anyone invested in their health to see what a portion size actually looks like for different foods. I often find myself exclaiming, "that's a serving size?" Especially on higher calorie foods such as peanut butter, mayonnaise, nuts, etc., it can be super helpful to have a visual example of the calorie content of different foods based on weight and volume!

I have carried a water bottle around with me ever since high school. Once I became aware of the environmental and physiological impact that plastics can have, I switched to stainless steel to avoid BPAs and I use a reusable container. I always notice a huge difference in my energy, satiety, mental focus, and even skin clarity when I have water accessible to me at all times. People often don't attribute issues such as a persistent appetite, low energy, or poor focus with being thirsty or dehydrated, but oftentimes water is the answer! I say, try drinking the recommended 2–3 liters of water a day and carry a water bottle around with you and see the difference it can make!

What are some typical challenges that your vegan clients experience, and how would you recommend addressing them?

I have heard a variety of responses from clients who have transitioned to a vegan diet, and the diversity is largely dependent on whether a vegan lifestyle is a good fit for the individual. Transitioning into a vegan diet does take diligent planning and attention to ensure a diverse and balanced diet.

Some clients talk about how full and satiated they feel and how much more energy they have. Others have described how they feel gassy, bloated, and low in energy. This is where listening to your body really makes the difference in determining if a vegan lifestyle is best for you.

Some of the most common challenges I hear my clients experience are:
- Struggling to find options when eating out
- Getting bored and eating the same things repetitively
- Eating bland food
- Missing variety
- Struggling with negative responses from peers, friends, and family members

To which my advice would be:
- Research the restaurants you are going to ahead of time by looking up their menu on line. Most places will have vegan options explicitly labeled and, if not, try and find something that can be "vegan-ified" such as sandwiches substituted with a veggie burger or avocado, salads with beans or tofu, or pasta with veggies and olive oil. I also recommend learning to get comfortable asking for substitutions. Some people can get panicky and feel embarrassed asking for special requests but I promise you that restaurants get hundreds of modifications on orders, so, there's no need to feel embarrassed!
- Have fun looking up vegan and plant-based foodie blogs online! There are thousands of passionate vegans who love to share the delicious recipes that they spend their time creating! Some of my favorites are Minimalist Baker, and Oh She Glows.

There are so many fun resources online to help keep things interesting!

·   I think finding a few food blogs or online resources can help with this, too, but learning how to use spices and marinades, and making a variety of dressings and dips, will help with keeping foods flavorful. The foundational foods of a vegan diet can be bland at first, but learning how to dress things up with toppings will always make your food delicious!

·   I find that getting inspired in the kitchen helps when you are missing variety. There is a substitution for literally every animal-based product to keep things interesting. Take a trip with some of your friends to the grocery store and try to find as many vegan products as you can! Sometimes, just learning what is available to you will help you feel like you have more options for variety!

·   This can be a big bummer, especially if you are the only one that eats differently amongst your peers, friends, or family members. Try to remember that you can never force others to change their behaviors, but you can try to explain how their behaviors impact you. I recommend that you have a strong internal motivation for why you are making the transition to a vegan lifestyle and then come up with a few responses that explain your decision in a positive light. Example might be, "I want to take better care of my body and a vegan lifestyle seems like an appealing way to do so" or "I feel great eating this way, and it seems to work great for my body." However, be aware that sometimes people choose to be negative regardless of your attitude. In these situations, remember that someone else's hostility or negativity is never about you and always about something they are struggling with internally!

What is the worst advice you hear people give routinely in the nutrition community?

In general, I think any advice that doesn't take into account your individuality is bad advice. Any change you make has to make sense for your own unique body as we are all so different and complex!

What is good advice for someone who is trying to lose weight?

There are a handful of factors that will make weight loss easier for most individuals which include:

1. Drinking plenty of water. Dehydration and thirst can sometimes feel like hunger or can make you feel "snacky", so drinking 2–3 liters of water throughout the day can absolutely help with satiety.
2. increasing your fiber intake from fruits and vegetables. When trying to lose weight, it's time to shift your thinking around about what will fill you up by focusing on eating as many fruits and vegetables as possible. Not only are these extremely beneficial for the body as sources of vitamins and minerals, but fresh fruits and vegetables also contain loads of fiber which helps you feel more satiated and keeps your digestive system functioning properly!
3. Increasing your protein at meals and snacks. Protein should be a priority at meals and snacks! Protein is an amazing tool for weight loss in that it literally shuts off hormones that make you feel hunger while boosting other hormones that make you feel full! If you feel hungry all of the time and feel like you are constantly eating, try increasing your protein to 20–30 grams at meal times and 10–15 grams at snacks and see how you feel!
4. Eat out less often. Excess calories from cooking oils, unhealthy preparation methods, added sugars and preservatives, and huge portion sizes almost always lead us to consume more than we actually need when eating out. Instead of focusing on the negative aspects of eating out less often, reconfigure your thinking to focus on the positives such as saving money, being more likely to accomplish your health-related goals, and having more control over the quality of your food by eating food you prepare at home! There's no need to miss out on the excitement or social aspects of eating out if you invite your friends over for a potluck or dinner at your house!

When patients come to see you for nutritional advice, what are some things they hear that usually surprise them?

One of the most common transitions I help my clients make is unlearning outdated advice based on old science or habits from their upbringing. This happens with everyone because we oftentimes get accidentally complacent to new information regarding nutrition and health. For everything, sticking with the most minimally processed option is almost always going to be your best bet. Ignore the label claims about "low-calories," "guilt-free," etc., and instead focus on eating as minimally processed as possible.

In the past few years, what attitude or belief has most shaped your understanding of healthy nutrition and a healthy lifestyle?

As most nutrition professionals have experienced, most of us come out of our academic education with an idea of how everyone should eat. However, I think you would be hard-pressed to find a nutrition professional who has not changed their paradigm regarding nutrition once they have worked with a lot of clients or patients. Soon enough, we all learn that bodies are all so different and taking the time to get to know the individual and listen to their experience is of upmost importance. Ignoring this step does a disservice to the individual! Personally, I think a healthy lifestyle requires the following: diversity in experiences so that you may grow intellectually, a love of fruits and vegetables so you can experience longevity, more smiles than frowns so you can experience bliss, and more friends than foes so that you can experience community.

Laura Kopec

Laura received a Master of Science in Health and Nutrition Education from Hawthorn University, a Master of Arts from the University of Arizona, a Doctorate in Traditional Naturopathy and a Nutritional Counseling Certificate from Trinity School of Natural Health. She is recognized by the American Alternative Medical Association as a Board Certified Alternative Medical Practitioner, and by the American Association of Drugless Practitioners as a board certified Holistic Health Practitioner.

Laura is dedicated to inspiring change and transformation in the lives of women and children everywhere. She is dedicated to the education, health, and wellness of women of all walks of life. Laura will help you reach your health and wellness goals and the health and wellness goals of your children. More information can be found on her website, laurakopec.com.

Top quote

"We do not realize how necessary proteins are to mental health."

What book about nutrition do you frequently recommend to friends?

Let's Get Real about Eating. I wrote that book because there was no guidebook to help people know the facts in simple form, and know how to strategize and take basic steps.

What are some typical challenges that your vegan clients experience, and how would you recommend addressing them?

When I visit with a client who has been living with a vegan diet, I often see imbalances in their mental health such as anxiety and depression. We do not realize how necessary proteins are to mental health, not just muscles, as often assumed. Secondly, I see the consequences of a high carbohydrate diet or sugar addictions, because often vegans are eating far too many simple and refined carbohydrates. These can also be mood related, but there can also be a weak digestion or weak immune system.

What is good advice for someone who is trying to lose weight?

I recommend my book, *The Linked Diet*, because there is so much misinformation and misconceptions surrounding diets and because, if someone does not change their mindset and address the real reasons they are overweight, weight loss will either not come or be fleeting.

When patients come to see you for nutritional advice, what are some things they hear that usually surprise them?

My clients are most often surprised to hear their symptoms originate in their stomach, and how the body works together as an entire system, and how telling their bowel movements are to their digestive system or their overall health. Our body tells us what is out of balance, but we have not been educated to understand this kind of body talk.

Kevin Kuhn

Kevin is a kinesiologist and sport nutrition coach. He has experience with athletic and non-athletic populations, and works primarily with youth athletes and endurance athletes looking to improve their physical performance, increase their adaptations to training, improve their body composition, improve their relationship with food, improve their health, and increase or decrease body weight. He has degrees in Exercise Science and Exercise Physiology with a focus on Nutritional Biochemistry.

Top quote

"The body is very well equipped to remove things that are toxic."

What book about nutrition do you frequently recommend to friends?

Layne Norton's book, *Fat Loss Forever,* is an excellent explanation of why "dieting" fails on a physiological level, psychological level, and sociological level. Any diet can be utilized to lose weight, and yet 95 percent of these diets are unsuccessful at maintaining weight loss. This book explains the how and why of this issue, and then provides strategies, behaviors, and methods for healthy weight loss and, most importantly, maintenance of weight loss.

How much does diet really affect mood and psychological well-being?

The question is, can you really be "hangry?" The exact amount will vary from person to person, but the evidence is very clear that both calorie load and macro/micronutrient breakdown have a profound effect on mood. Some markers of psychological stress and anxiety have been closely linked to blood glucose (blood sugar) levels dropping in circulation. Eating a snack or meal that helps to correct blood glucose levels, and aims to keep them steady, can have significant effects on mood, feelings of well-being, and focus.

Is the vegan diet equally good for everyone?

The answer to this question is highly dependent on the definition of "good." I view things through the lens of human movement and athletic performance, so, from my perspective, I do not believe this type of diet is equally good for everyone. Due to the adaptive differences between people living in vastly differing climates and locations, I believe some people are better adapted to eating a vegan or plant-based diet, while others are better adapted to a non-vegan or meat-based diet. Humans have teeth and digestive systems that have evolved to efficiently and effectively utilize both plant and animal sources of calories. That being said, I think everyone gains health benefits and perhaps even performance benefits from increasing plant-based foods in their diet. I think this may not be a very useful question.

A more useful question is what type of diet can you adhere to? People's dietary preferences vary greatly, so, trying to eat according to a specific diet may be an impossible task. If you believe you can eat plant-based today, tomorrow, next month, next year, and the rest of your life, then by all means follow a vegan diet. If you believe this will be an incredible struggle and an impossible task, then why set yourself up for failure? The majority of our health problems in modern society stem from a combination of too many calories and not enough activity. Any diet an individual can adhere to long-term is the most important priority when it comes to health and wellness.

From there, the next priority is to determine your body's calorie needs and stay consistently in that range. Any type of diet, even a vegan diet, that places you in either a chronic calorie surplus or chronic calorie deficit will eventually result in negative health outcomes. The vegan diet is a good diet if you can stick to it consistently, hit your calorie needs, hit your macronutrient needs (protein, fat, carbs), and hit your micronutrient needs (vitamins and minerals).

What are the top dangers of veganism, and how would you recommend avoiding them?

Again, my perspective is through the lens of optimal athletic performance. From this perspective, the potential limitations (not necessarily dangers) of veganism come from one primary area. This area is protein quality and quantity. If your goal is to maximize athletic adaptations to physiological stressors, i.e., become more athletic, then maximizing a positive nitrogen balance and maximally stimulating the synthesis of new muscle protein is key. This is important because without the synthesis of new muscle protein, the body cannot repair and recover from the stress of training, which means little to no adaptation (improvement in fitness) can occur.

When it comes to protein quality, the amino acids responsible for the synthesis of new muscle protein tend to be found in higher concentrations in animal-source protein in comparison to plant-source protein. The most important amino acid for muscle protein synthesis is the amino acid Leucine. The average person needs about three grams of Leucine to maximally stimulate the synthesis of new muscle protein. This can be reached by ingesting about 25–30 grams of whey protein, since whey is the protein source with the highest concentration of amino acid Leucine.

Plant-based sources of protein often contain about half the amount of Leucine per gram in comparison to animal-based protein sources, so, in order to maximize the synthesis of new muscle protein from plant-based protein sources, 45–55 grams of plant-based protein would need to be ingested. This is the limitation. Hitting not only a high daily protein goal (around 1 gram of protein per pound of body weight per day), but also chunking protein into a bolus (45+ grams per meal or snack) that is high enough to maximally stimulate protein synthesis, is extremely important for the plant-based athlete. This is not an impossible task. I work with many athletes who eat a plant-based diet who are able to hit these numbers and train and compete at an elite level.

Three big meals or seven small meals?

The answer to this question is answered by another question. "What can you adhere to long-term?" If three big meals fits your lifestyle and dietary preferences and, in turn, allows you to hit your calorie needs, macronutrient needs, and micronutrient needs, then stick with that. If you need smaller meals in order to consistently hit your calorie needs, macronutrient needs, and micronutrient needs, then go with that. Since adherence is the most important priority, it doesn't matter how many meals, as long as you are consistently doing whatever you have to do to hit the rest of the priorities.

What purchase of fifty dollars or less has improved your ability to have a healthy diet the most?

A tea-maker. I find it much easier to stay hydrated throughout the day if I have a pitcher of tea always available. Many people struggle to drink enough water throughout the day, so, this is one way to boost water intake while controlling other factors, like sugar intake. I like the taste of unsweetened tea, so, I don't typically add any sweeteners to my pitcher.

What are the two foods you'd recommend to stop eating or drastically cut out?

I hate to demonize any particular type of food, since I think everything in moderation is best, but I try to avoid hydrogenated oils and trans fats.

What is the worst advice you hear people give routinely in the nutrition community?

The worst advice I hear deals with anyone saying they have the specific diet that will help everyone. Any "one size fits all" approach or "everyone should eat this way" mentality is ideological and does not take into account individual differences in biochemistry, personal taste preferences, or lifestyle factors.

I think it is my job to say this as many times as is necessary: Find a diet or way of eating that you can stick to long term, then find out how many calories you need for optimal health, then set up your macronutrients so you can hit your calorie goal and reach your health and fitness goals, then eat a variety of foods so you can hit your micronutrient goals. You are unique, so, you're diet should be uniquely programmed for you.

What's the top "superfood" or supplement that you would recommend everyone should incorporate into their diet?

I think most people should eat more protein and fiber. There are plenty of high quality and inexpensive sources of both protein and fiber supplements on the market.

What is detoxification and how do you feel about the need for it?

Detoxification is the process by which the body removes toxins it views as harmful to the body. There is rarely, if ever, a need to "do a detox" or "cleanse" since the body is already very well equipped to remove things that are toxic. Anything the body views as a "toxin" that makes it through digestion and into the blood stream is transported through the blood stream to the liver. Here the toxin is converted from a fat-soluble state into a water-soluble state so that it can be flushed out of the body via sweat, urine, or other body fluids. It is extremely important to note that the flushing step cannot occur without adequate and consistent hydration and dietary protein intake. This is important since most "detoxes" focus on carbohydrate-rich fruit juice or nutrient dense vegetable juice, but very little protein.

Toxins that do not make it through the digestive process (into the blood stream) and therefore remain in the intestines are eliminated through waste, so, ensuring you eat enough dietary fiber is key to maintaining the body's natural detox system. So, save your time and money, because the only real detox you need to worry about is getting enough protein, high fiber fruits and veggies, and plenty of water. Your body literally evolved to do the rest.

Breakfast or no breakfast?

It all depends on the individual, but you still need to follow the 4 priorities: 1. adherence; 2. hitting your calorie needs; 3. hitting your macronutrient needs; and 4. hitting your micronutrient needs. If you can do all of that without having breakfast, and it fits your lifestyle so you can adhere to it long-term, then do that. If you need breakfast in order to hit your priorities, then eat breakfast.

In the past few years, what new attitude or belief has most shaped your understanding of healthy nutrition and a healthy lifestyle?

Perhaps the idea that even though everyone's biochemistry follows the same rules, there is enough variation and adaptation in our preferences and evolution that there is no "one way" when it comes to the human diet. We have specific calorie and macro/micro needs, but there are an infinite number of ways to address these needs. Forcing people to hit these needs by way of one specific diet is a sure-fire way to set up many people for failure.

What do you do when craving junk food?

When you are craving something, then, within reason and moderation, enjoy it. If that allows you to better maintain long-term adherence, then you are actually doing yourself a favor. If you go overboard with it and are unable to hit the rest of your priorities, then figure out what you may have to not eat in order to hit your priorities. Remove morality from food choices and focus on hitting your four main priorities. You will end up with fewer cravings because your mind won't fixate on the things it "can't" have based on arbitrary rules we subject ourselves to. Avoiding foods we crave can often result in binging, which can be much worse for your health than a reasonable treat within the framework of the four main priorities.

Komal Singh

Komal is an experienced nutritionist with a history of working in the health and wellness industry. She is skilled in nutritional counseling for weight management, diabetes, and hypertension. Komal has a Master's Degree in Nutrition, and an undergraduate degree in biochemistry and microbiology. She has been practicing for over ten years.

Top quote

"One needs to be in tune with one's body to understand the signals it gives. Your nutritional requirements and dietary habits need to change in the different phases of your life."

What purchase of fifty dollars or less has improved your ability to have a healthy diet the most?

It's not fifty dollars but I have always had a Braun multi-quick countertop hand blender with which I can easily chop vegetables, herbs, and nuts, and also blend vegetables for soups, and shred vegetables for salads, making it easier for me to use loads of vegetables in various forms in my meals, making them healthier.

What are some typical challenges that your vegan clients experience, and how would you recommend addressing them?

One of the main challenges my vegan clients generally face (besides the nutritional deficiencies) is social acceptance in terms of their food choices from family and friends, where most of them encounter initial resistance. However, it generally seems only to be a matter of time, and then people around them are either supportive or at least accept their decision.

What is worst advice you hear people give routinely in the nutrition community?

Advocating fad diets. Keto, for instance.

What is good advice for someone who is trying to lose weight?

My approach to good health and weight loss is holistic. So, besides cutting out processed foods, I believe in including whole and natural foods. One has to pay attention to one's emotional health, with sleep and exercise being equally important.

When patients come to see you for nutritional advice, what are some things they hear that usually surprise them?

Yes, a lot of my female clients especially are surprised by the fact that I recommend that they eat more food than they are currently eating because a lot of them go through a severe calorie restriction or they omit certain food groups completely. That leads to missing out or creating an imbalance of key nutrients. For instance, a lot of them omit nuts, eggs, or fruits like bananas, with the perception that these are fattening. So, including nutrient-dense foods which are wholesome and natural brings about positive changes in their overall health along with weight loss.

When it comes to weight loss, most people are so hyper-focused on the little stuff that they cannot see how restrictive they are being. Some of the common misconceptions are avoiding healthy foods like bananas, mangoes, and nuts with the notion that these are "fattening." Or people completely eliminate grains and skip meals only to replace them with highly processed energy or protein bars. Being on self-imposed restrictive diets based on food fear and not facts leads them to not being in a state of optimal health and well being and may also bring around frustration.

So, during my consultations, when I bust the myths and advocate liberalizing foods based on their nutrient requirements, and achieving an overall balance, some women are amazed. The look on the client's face when they say, wait, I can eat all of that? is a beautiful moment!

In the past few years, what attitude or belief has most shaped your understanding of healthy nutrition and a healthy lifestyle?

In my experience, I have understood that each individual is different and nutrition requirements will vary according to factors like health issues and goals that need to be addressed. One needs to be in tune with one's body to understand the signals it gives. Your nutritional requirements and dietary habits need to change in different phases of your life. Besides nutrition, a holistic approach to reduce stress, staying active, and good quality sleep are very important. Incorporating diet and exercise habits which are sustainable is of more value. Achieving a lifestyle with a balance in emotional and physical health is key to well being.

Elissa Goodman

Elissa Goodman is one of LA's premiere cleanse experts and holistic nutritionists. After being diagnosed with cancer when she was thirty-two, Elissa explored holistic alternatives and combined them with traditional treatments and was able to beat the disease. She is the author of the S.O.U.P cleanse and multiple books on the subject.

Elissa's mission is to educate and encourage healthy, mindful living while helping others to embrace the concept that we are a product of what we eat and how we treat ourselves. This health warrior has helped countless people navigate their way through the daunting world of Cancer treatments and the healing process.

Top quote

"The truth is that food is medicine."

What purchase of fifty dollars or less has improved your ability to have a healthy diet the most?

The unplug app for meditation!

What is the worst advice you hear people give routinely in the nutrition community?

There are a few recurring themes, as far as the worst advice.

First, eating animal protein at every meal is a big problem, and a myth. Some people say this satiates you more so. That's just not true, and is a real problem.

Second, the carb-free diet is also a big problem, because it's hard to sustain and people miss out on key nutrients.

Then, there's any form of extreme dieting. We need to get all different types of veggies and foods in our diet to get all the nutrients and vitamins that we need. To overdo any one of them is no good. Even overdoing something "healthy" like kale isn't good.

Neglecting emotions and living in an emotionally healthy way is the big ticket to success with healthy eating habits and any health. And it can create a vicious cycle because following some protocol creates more stress.

Low-fat vs. low-carb diet for weight loss?

I produce a program in Los Angeles that I deliver to over 100 people a month. It's soups, tonics, lattes, bars, etc.

Both low-fat and low-carb are bogus. My program has a lot of legumes, beans, quinoa, healthy fats, and healthy complex carbs. I am not into restriction. We all know that simple carbs are bad, and bad fats are bad, but everything in moderation is important. Fats satiate you, they rev up your metabolism. Carbs calm you down and make you feel less anxious.

The whole keto philosophy is a very difficult way to maintain your weight. I don't like anything too restrictive. It could be great for the short term and for certain ailments, but it's not something you can sustain. You're not getting enough minerals to calm your body down.

I've seen people who go on low-carb diets become anxious and have trouble sleeping. They usually don't do well.

In the past few years, what attitude or belief has most shaped your understanding of healthy nutrition and a healthy lifestyle?

The truth is that food is medicine. For me, it's going back to the basics of eating real food. How can you go wrong with that? The food that was put on this planet was put on the planet for a reason. Eating the foods that we know instinctively that are going to elevate our health is good. Plants and vegetables. More of a plant-based diet with a little of animal protein, not a lot.

What is crucial these days is that for all of us to be always the healthiest that we can be is that we have to tap into our instincts. Every one of us knows what the right thing is to eat. We know how we feel when we eat the wrong thing, and we know how we feel when we eat the right thing.

It's about trusting yourself and learning how foods make you feel and following and trusting your instincts further. We are all emotional and we have these emotional reasons for eating.

When we are stressed, we are living out of body. We are living in a fight-or-flight mode. When we are in that place, it's hard to figure out what is right for you and what isn't right for you. You're not able to listen to that instinct, your "gut," so, it's very important to get into the right stress-free mindset.

One book I like is *Radical Remission*. It is about how cancer victims dealt with their stress, the toxic relationships in their lives, and all that emotional baggage. That always sits pretty heavy with people and affects many aspects of their lives.

The most important thing that I've learned about the journey of getting myself into remission is the idea of taking a step back and truly loving myself. We're always told that to feel good about ourselves and to love ourselves is selfish. We're trained in that mindset, which is actually the opposite of having a healthy life.

When people ask you, "do you really love yourself," most people come up with excuses and not all the beautiful things about ourselves. We've been trained to not focus on that. It's always like, "I wish I was skinnier, had more money, better relationships, etc." None of that is really important. You can love yourself just because it's you, and you are worth loving, and your heart is something that should be cherished and really taken care of.

If we don't really go there, then we won't take the time to make the choices about health that matter. The comparison mindset (keeping up, feeling we're not good enough) creates a sense of anxiety that prevents you from feeling calm, sleeping better, and having depression, and not being in touch with your true appetite.

If you just surrender to the fact that you deserve the things you want, you will get them.

This is a little hard to do on your own. Over the years, I've investigated people who can release those thought patterns. There's so many people out there doing this and so many ways! Meditation, psychologists, people who can work with energy well.

How do you find such a good person? There are a lot of people who can do harm actually. First of all, you need to trust your instincts. Do you have a good feeling about this person? Find out if they are willing to work with you based on what you really want or if they have some inflexible agenda. Finding a good one is tricky! I've used about ten in my life, and about three were really good.

The important thing is to release energy. The bottom line is that your subconscious is quite full by the age of seven. It really is a lot of subconscious thinking that is what I'm talking about. The patterns and negative things that happened in the early days, and you're just repeating those memories and mindset. Anything that can actually release, shake things up, release anxiety, negativity, etc., is really important and helpful. Whether it's tapping techniques, breathing exercises, intense massages, primal scream therapy, etc., all of that is useful!

What is your morning routine?

My morning routine is simple. I wake up and drink 16 ounces of water. Then I meditate for 15–20 minutes and I might use Unplugged App. Then I make a cup of coffee with collagen powder and MCT oil. After that, I make a green juice (without any fruits, because of the sugar). During that time, I'm already on the computer or phone! I basically try for the first 30–60 minutes not to jump right into it.

Keri Gans

Keri Gans is a Registered Dietitian Nutritionist, Certified Yoga Teacher, spokesperson and media personality based in New York City. She is the author of *The Small Change Diet*, a Shape Magazine Advisory Board Member, and blogger for US News & World Report.

Keri is frequently quoted in local and national publications such as Glamour, Fitness, Shape, Self, Women's Health, and US News. She is a sought-after nutrition expert on television and her appearances include The Dr. Oz Show, ABC News, PIX11 Morning Show, Primetime, Good Morning America, and FOX Business.

Top quote

"Nighttime snacking for the average person means they are consuming calories they don't need."

What book about nutrition do you frequently recommend to friends?

I don't typically don't recommend books. If you're going to read a book about nutrition, I would recommend that it's written by a registered dietician or Ph.D. I don't recommend books about nutrition written by celebrities, or individuals looking to promote products, or books that promote the elimination of certain food groups (carbs, dairy). I feel that those are red flags.

Is the vegan diet equally good for everyone?

That is a very tough question.

I think, first of all, you need to know the reason someone is choosing a vegan diet. For people who have a history of eating disorders, they could be looking for an excuse to restrict their food.

If someone has a medical condition such as diabetes, it's not that it's not possible but I'm concerned that an individual with diabetes gets adequate protein with every meal. It's not that it's not possible with every diet. If an individual doesn't like the options present in a vegan diet, it's harder to meet those needs. So, I'd be more concerned.

It could be good for everyone, but it depends on a person's likes and dislikes food wise. If someone doesn't like tofu/tempeh/satin, I'd be concerned. I've found that working with many individuals, they were picky eaters. If those picky eaters go vegan, it's hard to meet their needs. If the picky eater is a diabetic, then I'd be totally against a vegan lifestyle.

Even if people follow the vegan diet carefully, I would not say that a vegan diet is going to be necessarily better than a flexitarian diet. Another important component is whether the diet makes you happy. That's important!

If you're going to practice a vegan diet, it is a lifestyle. I don't want to see leather shoes or a leather jacket on you.

What are the top risks of a vegan diet that you've seen, and how would you recommend avoiding them?

First risk, efficiency of B12. If you're not consuming animal products, you're not consuming B12. To prevent a B12 deficiency, a vegan must supplement. It would be smart for a vegan to get their B12 levels checked.

Second risk, calcium. Vegans will claim that you can get enough calcium from dark green leafy vegetables, and from foods that have been fortified. However, you need a lot. It's not that it's not possible, it's just a little harder. You need around five cups of broccoli to equal one cup of milk. So it's possible, but you have to really eat enough or you have to supplement.

Third risk, vitamin D. Vitamin D is a problem for many to begin with. Fish, bones, fortified milk, all these contain vitamin D. Vitamin D is also critical for calcium absorption.

Fourth risk, being a picky eater. If you're a picky eater, it's hard to meet all the needs such as protein, iron, etc.

Fifth risk, if you have a history of eating disorders, make sure you're not using a vegan diet as an excuse to restrict what you eat. I've seen that a lot in my practice. I find it more so in younger women because a lot of times it becomes about weight. If someone choses to be vegan because they are older and they have a history of heart disease, it's one thing. But, if it's about weight, then it could be a red flag. It totally depends on the individual.

Three big meals or seven small meals?

There is no one set rule. I don't support either! If I had to chose between the two, I'd choose breakfast, lunch, dinner, and a snack in between. The average person probably shouldn't be eating after dinner, because that's usually a habit. If the dinner would be well-balanced enough, and if they aren't staying up too late, it shouldn't be an issue.

When we talk about diet, there's nothing that is 100 percent true for everyone. Nighttime snacking for the average person means they are consuming calories they don't need. For the average person, it becomes the excess of something and, given the state of our society, for most people it's too many calories!

What are the two foods you'd recommend to stop eating or drastically cut out?

I don't recommend any foods to drastically cut out. There are foods that we should eat more of and and foods we should eat less off, but the mentality that we should eliminate something isn't the best. It's too drastic of a mindset!

For example, I would question someone who is regularly drinking soda. I would question why? But if someone came to me said, "I'm not giving up one Coke a day," I'd figure out how we could get enough healthy foods into them! But I wouldn't cut out the Coke.

We should be able to enjoy our foods and not fear them. There are no bad or good foods. I believe there are foods that are better for you and we should eat them. On occasion, any food can be good if it makes you happy.

Likewise, no food can be a "silver bullet" in our diet. We need to look at what people eat over the course of a week, and not zero onto "one food" or "one mineral" and look at the overall picture. Even if someone eats one hotdog a week, if they are getting enough fruits or vegetables, that's what I would be focused on.

What is worst advice you hear people give routinely in the nutrition community?

"Shop the perimeter." That's the belief that the outer isles of the supermarket are what you want. That's wrong because you're missing the beans, the legumes, etc. We should encourage people to shop the entire supermarket, but with a plan. I'm more concerned that people have a shopping list, and that list should bring people to the center of the supermarket for the quinoa, the whole grains, the nuts, etc.!

We have too many things about detoxes. Anytime I hear that we need to detox, it should be taken with a grain of salt. Our bodies naturally detox ourselves every single day! You don't need to go on a detox to do that. What you need to do is eat a healthy diet and you then won't need to go on a detox. That means not eating an overall super processed diet, high sugar diet, fried fat foods, the chips, the greasy fries. If your diet is of that caliber, no wonder you feel like you need to do something drastic. You need to make better healthier choices, more 100 percent whole foods, and you will probably feel better.

If certain foods make you sleep better or less, that's important. If something disrupts your sleep, that can play a role but it's not clear if it's the actual food or the sleep.

Low-fat vs. low-carb diet for weight loss?

Portion control for weight loss! Low fat didn't work because people replaced it with even more calories. Low carb doesn't work because their portions of protein are too big.

The arguments that low carb lowers insulin is very individual. For some, it doesn't work. Is it for diabetic control, for weight loss, what is the goal? It's highly personalized and it's important to keep that in mind. Everyone is slightly different and what works best for one person, won't work well for someone else.

The best diet is when someone is at their best. They are happy and have a healthy relationship with food, their labs are normal (blood sugar, cholesterol, etc.), they sleep well, and they have energy.

Breakfast or no breakfast?

It depends on what your end game is. Research will state that perhaps eating breakfast doesn't play into weight loss. (The "it's the important meal of the day.") I'm still in support of breakfast, because it's an opportunity for certain nutrients for the rest of the day. If we're talking weight loss, whichever you prefer. If we're talking getting nutrients, it's a great opportunity to get some of those nutrients.

Depending on how old you are, research also supports that you concentrate better after you've eaten a breakfast (at least in children, and it's not hard to believe that that's true for adults). So that also plays into it!

Coffee on an empty stomach affects some people, others it doesn't. If it makes you jittery or gives any GI distress, then no, but it doesn't have that effect on everyone.

In the past few years, what attitude or belief has shaped your understanding of healthy nutrition and a healthy lifestyle the most?

One thing we can count on is that science is constantly evolving. Just because a new study comes out and states X, that doesn't mean we have to change things. Just look at eggs. They were bad for us, then they became good for us. Now, the latest study claims eggs are bad again. However, when you dive deeply, the information was taken as a diet recall. Diet recall isn't the most reliable.

There is no one diet that's for everyone. When we talk about healthy nutrient and lifestyle, it has to be sustainable. In order to be a healthy individual, it has to be a lifestyle commitment. It includes what's on our plate but it also includes how we sleep and also how active we are. It's not just one factor.

What do you do when you're craving junk food?

I don't really crave junk food. If I do, I eat it. Too many people don't allow into their diets the foods they crave. If they did, perhaps they'd have better control of them.

I've had too many women who go out drinking and what happens when they stay out late is that they eat a lot of pizza. What works better is to allow yourself a slice here and there. Incorporate them in some way into your diet, and you'll crave them less and less. Again, it all comes back to developing a healthy relationship with all foods. Even the foods you crave that are junk. Nutrition is an evolving science because the data is changing. Where there were some uncertainties before, science has started to extrapolate.

Lolin Hilgartner

Lolin received her Bachelors of Science degree in Kinesiology from the University of Maryland. She was trained at Western States Chiropractic College in Portland, Oregon and became a Chiropractic Physician in 1993. She has had extensive training in nutrition and functional Medicine and is a Certified Nutritional Specialist by the American College of Nutrition. Her areas of particular interest are treating children with behavioral or attention issues, addressing immune issues of all kinds including natural treatments for Lyme Disease, and restoring gut health.

Dr. Hilgartner, along with her husband, Dr. Pete Hilgartner, has been in practice in Leesburg, Virginia for over twenty-five years.

Top quote

"I see vegans eating a lot of breads and cereals and muffins and pancakes which, although tasty, are fairly deficient in nutrients, high in starches and carbs, and will lead a person in a short time down the diabetes path."

What book about nutrition do you frequently recommend to friends?

One of my favorite books for patients that I also have my staff and interns read is Weston Price's book, *Nutrition and Physical Degeneration*. He documents, both in text and with pictures, the marked changes that occur in the individual and also the community with the introduction of inferior diets, e.g., diets that contain less nutrients and/or more sugars.

Another favorite and a quick and easy read is Francis Pottenger's book, *Pottenger's Cats*. Dr. Pottenger did several extensive studies on cats. One study looked at cats and nutrients. With both a control group and an experimental group, he modified the food in the experimental group so that it was nutritionally inferior, and he observed what changes occurred in successive generations of cats.

Pottenger observed structural changes in the offspring such as narrowing of the face and pelvis, increased thyroid issues, changes in their skin and coat, increased illnesses, increased cancers, and shortening of lifespan. He also observed personality and behavioral changes. Eventually they experienced fertility issues and could no longer reproduce. I believe we are seeing the same thing played out in our society today, with the fairly recent dependence on processed and fast foods.

What was most encouraging was that, when Pottenger started feeding the experimental cats nutritionally complete foods again, each generation became healthier until they once again resembled the control groups. I would like to see this taught in our schools, and I consistently share this information with my patients.

What purchase of fifty dollars or less has improved your ability to have a healthy diet the most?

I bought an enormous freezer for twenty-five dollars on Craig's List which enables me to stock up and freeze fruits and vegetables when fresh for consumption year round so I don't have to buy from other countries or pay premium prices in the winter. Most importantly, I don't have to run to the grocery store as often, which saves me tons of money and time and decreases the temptation to buy convenience-based, processed foods.

What are some typical challenges that your vegan clients experience, and how would you recommend addressing them?

First is staying vegan. Almost every vegan I know is cheating somewhere, eating butter or cheeses, milk, eggs or fish. These are very natural and healthy cravings because we need fats to live.

The second challenge I see with being or staying vegan is where are you getting your fat-soluble vitamins from? Your vitamins A, D, and E? Your EPA and DHA? These are critical to our health in so very many ways. Nowadays, you can get them from supplements but you have to pay careful attention to make sure you get high quality ones.

Additionally, most vegans are not eating that many vegetables. Vegetables are great for us, no doubt, but I see vegans eating a lot of breads and cereals and muffins and pancakes which, although tasty, are fairly deficient in nutrients, high in starches and carbs, and will lead a person in a short time down the diabetes path. Ingestion of omega-3's from fish or grass fed meat can turn off enzymes that lead to diabetes, so, not only are vegans eating a high carb diet (anything not a protein is a carb) but they are missing valuable fats that can help keep diabetes in check. Therefore, extra care must be taken to avoid diabetes and the symptoms of diabetes.

Another common challenge I see is inflammation associated with the vegan diet. Fats from plants are rich in omega-6's, which feed a pathway called the arachidonic acid pathway, which is a pro-inflammatory pathway. Omega-3's, rich in animal sources, are anti inflammatory and generally "put the fire out" with an anti-inflammatory diet.

Our body tries to keep a ratio of 1:2 of omega 3's to 6's in order to keep inflammation at bay. Without the use of animal sources, this can be challenging. Flax seed is a source of 3's, but also has significant 6's. The omega balance should be tested and followed as well as markers for inflammation. It is essential that other issues that may contribute to inflammation be addressed such as MTHFR status and blood sugar issues. Ingestion of healthy fats such as olive oil, sesame seed oil, borage, wheat germ, coconut, and palm oil is essential.

What is the biggest "wrong advice" that you hear regularly when it comes to vegan nutrition and a vegan lifestyle?

Protein shakes.

If they are whey based (animal based), they start out with cholesterol and when you dry liquid whey under high heat and temperatures, a byproduct called oxidized cholesterol is formed. This is what we feed to lab rabbits because it clogs their arteries right up and pharmaceutical companies then use them to test new drugs.

The food industry knows this is a dangerous byproduct of processing, and is quietly moving away from whey protein, so, we are now seeing an uptick in pea protein shakes.

Peas, being a plant, are incomplete proteins, meaning they don't have all the amino acids it takes to build muscle, so, the label should read, "Incomplete Protein Powder." Throwing a highly processed pea powder together with some synthetic vitamins is not and never will be a health food.

What is good advice for someone who is trying to lose weight?

Don't cut back calories. If you cut calories, you cut energy to your body much like only putting a gallon of gas in your car. This stresses your body and does not result in any long-term gain.

True weight loss occurs when we boost our metabolism. We want to run with a full tank of gas rather than a half tank of gas. So, we don't want to cut calories. We want calories that benefit our body, so, we will lose weight if we get our calories from nutrient-packed foods like liver pate or salads with olive oil and vinegar versus starchy processed foods.

I teach candida diets with my patients, individually and in groups, and this is a no-sugar diet. People eat 2,000 calories or more per day on the diet and, even though it's not a weight loss diet, everybody loses weight. Over a six week period, patients will experience 5–47 pound losses just by changing the TYPE of foods they are eating, not the amount of calories. This is not even a ketogenic diet. This is just what happens when we replace sugars and starches with nutrient-rich foods. So, a low glycemic index diet is key but this shouldn't be a "diet." This should be how we eat all the time.

We also need to look at an individual's metabolism, their individual makeup, and see if there are any stressors that are draining a body's resources. Thyroid, adrenal, blood sugar handling issues, infection, inflammation, irritable bowel disease, constipation, nutritional deficiencies, diarrhea, medications, antibiotic use, illnesses, genetic inheritance, and other things all create stress on the body that lowers the metabolism and leads to weight gain.

Some people gain weight because of poor food choices but, in my practice, most people have weight issues SECONDARY to health issues. Weight needs to be recognized as a sign of unwellness much like that of a fever, requiring a thorough clinical history and exam.

When patients come to see you for nutritional advice, what are some things they hear that usually surprise them?

I don't take my patients off of meat completely. Whereas I abhor conventional animal farming operations for the cruel and horrific way animals are treated, I believe we vote with our dollars. If you just stop eating meat, you are taking your dollar out of the game. To elicit change in large corporations, change your buying habits. This is much more effective than hoping for government regulations or for them to grow a conscience.

When corporations see that we are willing to spend a couple extra bucks to know that the animal we are having for dinner had a good healthy outside life, then they will want to provide the same thing in order to capture our dollar. We are already seeing this happening. Every large corporation is investing in organic foods and vitamin and supplement companies, etc., because they see where Americans are spending their money and they want a piece of it.

In the past few years, what attitude or belief has shaped your understanding of healthy nutrition and a healthy lifestyle the most?

When I started out in nutrition over twenty-five years ago, I thought that supplements were a tool to facilitate healing and to help restore health, but I did not consider them necessary for the long term.

I now give classes on toxins in our food, air, water, and homes. I see kids that are put on medications on the first day of their lives. I have patients getting cancer in their teens. I don't know a single person or patient that hasn't been on antibiotics at least once in their lives.

I know that newborn babies have hundreds of chemicals in them on the day they are born, including breakdown products of DDT which was banned forty-seven years ago.

Children consume an estimated 12 percent of their calories from fast food restaurants, meaning that 12 percent of their calories are harmful (trans fats, hydrogenated oils, preservatives, food dyes, stabilizers, etc.,) or at the very least, useless.

Americans eat about fifty million fast food meals per day, and the majority of other meals is processed foods. Our soils are polluted and devoid of minerals and most of our food arrives on a truck rather from our backyard.

So, I now believe that supplements are necessary, even CRITICAL, if one hopes to be healthy. I believe that there are many superfoods like cod liver oil, turmeric, spirulina and chlorella, and many nutrients like calcium, magnesium, zinc, and iodine which should be taken every day. One should try to find whole-food-based supplements because these are safe to take long term.

"Truth—more precisely, an accurate understanding of reality—is the essential foundation for producing good outcomes."

Ray Dalio